MW01673591

Get Healthy and Quit Smoking Natural Way

Quit Drinking and Smoking by Following Easy Steps to a Natural Healing and Living

Verda Estrada

Disclaimer and Terms of Use: Effort has been made to ensure that the information in this book is accurate and complete, however, the author and the publisher do not warrant the accuracy of the information, text and graphics contained within the book due to the rapidly changing nature of science, research, known and unknown facts and internet.

The Author and the publisher do not hold any responsibility for errors, omissions or contrary interpretation of the subject matter herein. This book is presented solely for motivational and informational purposes only.

Contents

INTRODUCTION 8

9+1 GUIDES TO QUIT SMOKING 31

1. CUTTING DOWN TO QUIT.................................34

2. COLD TURKEY 41

3. NICOTINE GUM..50

4. NICOTINE LOZENGE...60

5. TRANSDERMAL PATCH BUPROPION SUSTAINED RELEASE (SR) 64

6. VARENICLINE...69

7. TAKING NON NICOTINE MEDICATIONS........74

8. WEB-BASED/ON-LINE SUPPORT........................90

9. QUIT LINE 96

10. SUPPORT GROUPS..103

PROLOGUE 109

What you should know about Alcohol *112*

What are the different drinking levels?.......................... *113*

When is moderate drinking still too much? *114*

How Long Does Alcohol Stay In The Body? *116*

What is a standard drink?... *117*

How do you know how much alcohol is in your drink? 118

Women and Alcohol 120

WEEK ONE **124**

DAY ONE 125

DAY TWO 135

DAY THREE 139

DAY FOUR 143

DAY FIVE 147

DAY SIX 150

DAY SEVEN 155

WEEK TWO **157**

DAY EIGHT AND NINE 159

DAY TEN AND ELEVEN 163

DAY TWELVE AND THIRTEEN 166

DAY FOURTEEN 169

WEEK THREE **174**

DAY FIFTEEN TO TWENTY-ONE 178

WEEK FOUR **183**

DAY TWENTY-TWO TO TWENTY-FOUR 190

DAY TWENTY-FIVE AND TWENTY-SIX 197

DAY TWENTY-SEVEN AND TWENTY-EIGHT 206

INTRODUCTION: 211

HISTORY OF DRINKING..215

RISK FACTORS FOR ALCOHOLISM 228

THE EFFECTS OF PARENTAL ALCOHOLISM ON CHILDREN 233

FACTORS THAT CONTRIBUTE TO ALCOHOLISM 237

HOW CHILDREN OF ALCOHOLICS MIGHT REACT WHEN THEY'RE ANGRY..241

UNDERAGE DRINKING PROBLEM 247

QUITTING ALCOHOL..276

5 WAYS STOP DRINKING HAS AN EFFECT ON YOUR BRAIN 304

THE BEST MEDITATION TECHNIQUES FOR DRINKING ALCOHOL TODAY..................................310

WHAT CAUSES PEOPLE TO RELAPSE? 318

HISTORY OF SMOKING...340

THE EAST ASIAN REGION 354

SOCIAL STIGMATIZATION 356

Politics undergoing a renaissance 357

THE FOLLOWING COMPOUNDS ARE FOUND IN CIGARETTE SMOKE: 360

WHY IS IT SO HARD TO QUIT? 364

o Health risks can be reduced 367

THE MENTAL HEALTH OF SMOKERS MAY BE IMPROVED BY QUITTING 369

Nicotine and dopamine 372

Nicotine withdrawal lasts how long? 377

Withdrawal symptoms on the physical level ... 383

SYMPTOMS RELATING TO THE MIND, EMOTIONS, AND BEHAVIOR 387

The timeline for withdrawing from nicotine .. 388

WHY DO WOMEN CONTINUE TO SMOKE DURING PREGNANCY? 395

MOTIVATING INTERVENTIONS 420

BEST TIPS TO STOP SMOKING 433

Epilogue 450

Introduction

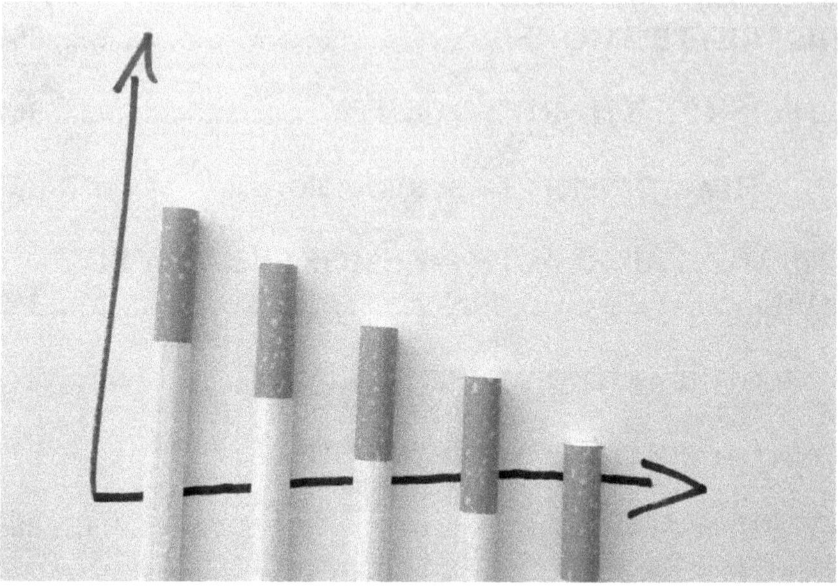

Around 6 trillion cigarettes are smoked worldwide every year .Although by and large utilization has declined marginally in the course of recent years, the future way of worldwide tobacco control is as yet dubious. Regardless of the logical responsibility of some in the tobacco business towards smoking world, all significant tobacco organizations proceed to forcefully publicize cigarettes and overwhelmingly battle tobacco control endeavors around the globe. The critical decreases in smoking rates in the United Kingdom, Australia, Brazil, and different nations that have executed the most developed tobacco control laws internationally are as a rule balance by the expanding utilization in numerous nations with more fragile tobacco control guidelines.

For a large part of the twentieth century, smoking was viewed as a socially scholarly propensity and as an individual decision. It is just in the previous decade or with the goal that the major part of nicotine in supporting smoking conduct has started to be all the more broadly acknowledged. It is currently perceived that cigarette smoking is essentially an appearance of nicotine enslavement and that smokers have independently trademark inclinations for their degree of nicotine admission. Smokers direct the manner in which they puff and breathe in to accomplish their ideal nicotine portion.

The connection with nicotine compulsion doesn't suggest that pharmacological elements drive smoking conduct in a basic manner and to the avoidance of different impacts. Social, monetary, individual, and political impacts all have a significant influence in deciding examples of smoking predominance and end. In spite of the fact that medication impacts support the conduct, family and more extensive social impacts are regularly basic in figuring out who starts smoking, who surrenders, and who proceeds.

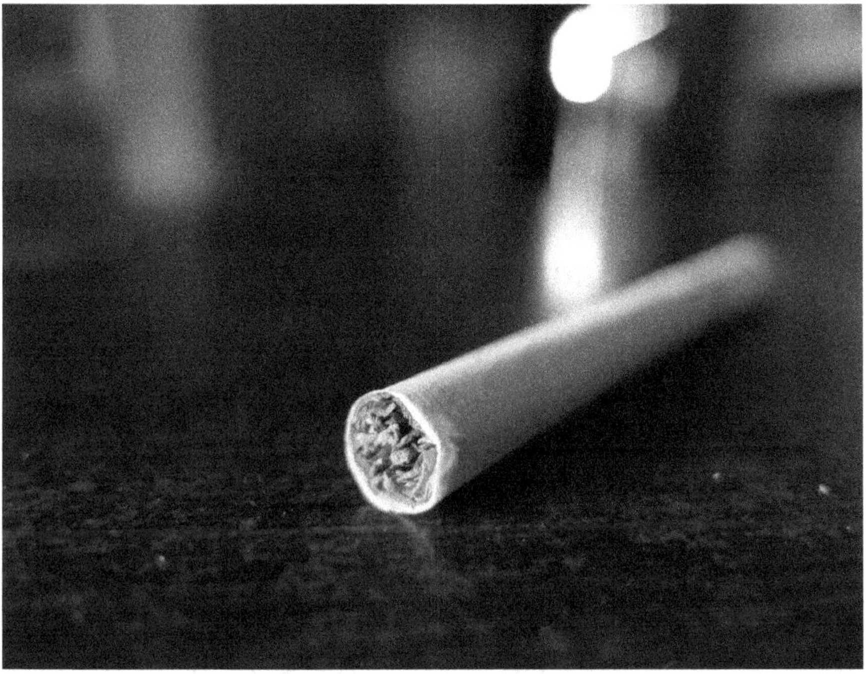

Why do people smoke?

The vast majority who smoke began smoking when they were youngsters. The individuals who have companions and additionally guardians who smoke are bound to begin smoking than the individuals who don't. A few teens say that they "simply needed to attempt it," or they thought it was "cool" to smoke.

The tobacco business' advertisements, value breaks, and different advancements for its items are a major impact in our general public. The tobacco and smoking business burns through billions of dollars every year to make and market promotions that show smoking as energizing, impressive, and safe. Tobacco use is additionally appeared in computer games, on the web, and on TV. What's more, motion pictures showing individuals smoking are another huge impact. Studies show that youngsters who see smoking in motion pictures are bound to begin smoking.

A fresher impact on tobacco use is the e-cigarette and other cutting edge, in vogue electronic "vamping" gadgets. Frequently wrongly seen as innocuous as and simpler to get and use than customary tobacco items, these gadgets are a route for new clients to figure out how to breathe in and get dependent on nicotine, which can set them up for smoking.

Trying different things with smoking normally happens in the early teen years and is driven overwhelmingly by psychosocial intentions. For a fledgling, smoking a cigarette is a representative demonstration passing on messages, for example, in the expressions of the tobacco organization Philip Morris, "I'm not, at this point my mom's youngster," and "I'm intense." Children who are pulled in to this juvenile declaration of saw adulthood or defiance will in general come from foundations that favor smoking (for instance, with undeniable degrees of smoking in guardians, kin, and companions; moderately denied neighborhoods; schools where smoking is normal). They likewise tend not to be prevailing as per their own or society's terms (for instance, they have low confidence, have disabled mental prosperity, are overweight, or are helpless achievers at school).

The ideal picture is adequate for the beginner smoker to endure the revolution of the initial not many cigarettes, after which pharmacological components accept a lot more prominent significance. Again in the expressions of Philip Morris, "as the power from the psychosocial imagery dies down, the pharmacological impact takes over to support the propensity." Within a year or so of beginning to smoke, kids breathe in a similar measure of nicotine per cigarette as grown-ups, experience desiring for cigarettes when they can't smoke, make endeavors to stop, and report encountering the entire scope of nicotine withdrawal manifestations.

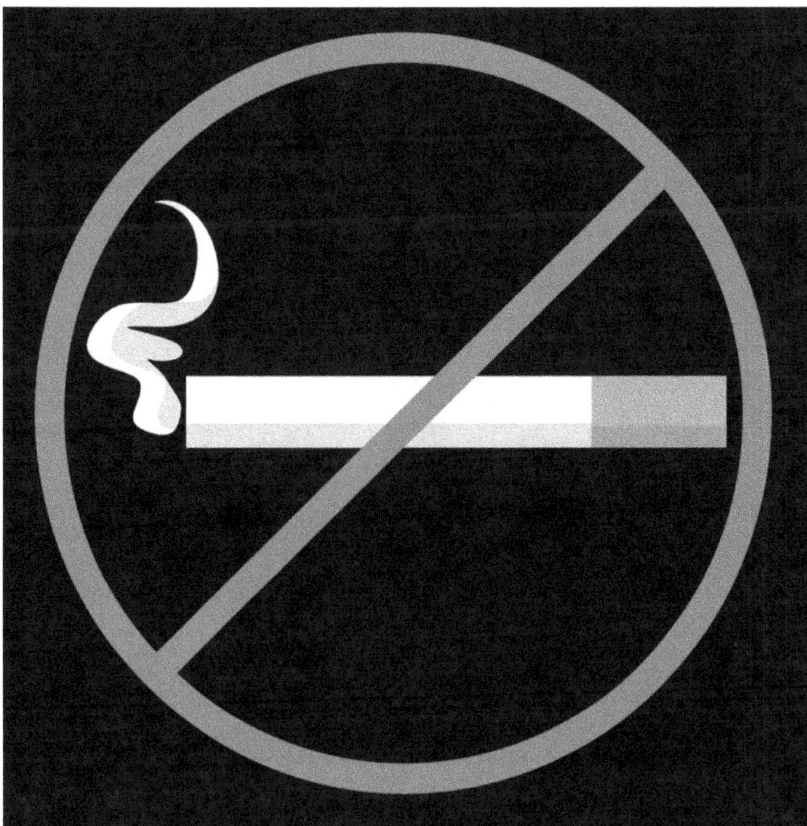

Any individual who starts utilizing tobacco can get dependent on nicotine. Studies show that smoking is well on the way to turn into a

propensity during the adolescent years. The more young and youthful you are when you start to smoke, the almost certain you are to get dependent on nicotine.

As indicated by a report almost 9 out of 10 grown-ups who smoke began before age 18, and essentially completely began by age 26. The report gauges that around 3 out of 4 secondary school smokers will become grown-up smokers regardless of whether they mean to stop in a couple of years.

Enslavement is set apart by the rehashed, impulsive chasing or utilization of a substance notwithstanding its hurtful impacts and undesirable outcomes. Enslavement is mental or passionate reliance on a substance. Nicotine is the known addictive substance in tobacco. Ordinary utilization of tobacco items prompts compulsion in numerous clients. Nicotine is a medication that happens normally in tobacco and it's believed to be just about as addictive as heroin or cocaine.

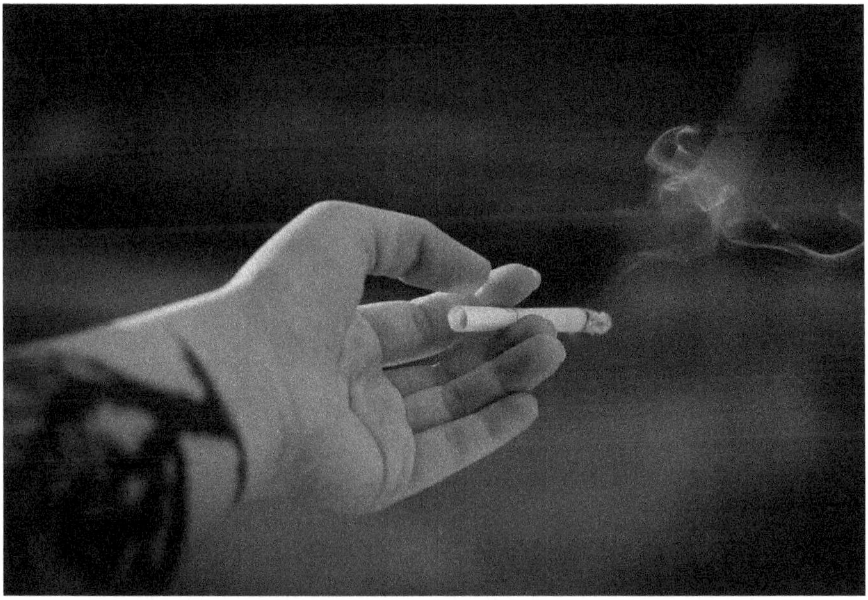

Effects of nicotine

- Nicotine and different synthetic substances in tobacco smoke are handily assimilated into the blood through the lungs. From that point, nicotine rapidly spreads all through the body.

- At the point when taken in limited quantities, nicotine causes charming emotions and occupies the client from undesirable sentiments. This makes the tobacco client need to utilize more. It follows up on the science of the cerebrum and focal sensory system, influencing temperament. Nicotine works a lot of like other irresistible medications, by flooding the cerebrum's prize circuits with a compound called dopamine. Nicotine additionally gives a tad of an adrenaline surge - adequately not to see, but rather enough to accelerate the heart and raise circulatory strain.
- Nicotine arrives at the cerebrum inside the space of seconds in the wake of enjoying a drag, and its belongings begin

to wear off inside a couple of moments. The client may begin to feel aggravated and restless. Generally it doesn't arrive at the purpose of genuine withdrawal side effects; however the individual utilizing the item gets more awkward over the long run. This is the thing that regularly drives the smoker to illuminate once more. Eventually, the individual uses tobacco, the unsavory sentiments disappear, and the cycle proceeds. In the event that the smoker doesn't smoke again soon, withdrawal manifestations deteriorate after some time.

- As the body adjusts to nicotine, individuals who use it will in general build the measure of tobacco they use. This raises the measure of nicotine in their blood, and more tobacco is expected to get a similar impact. This is called resistance. Over the long haul, a specific nicotine level is reached and the individual should keep up the utilization to keep the degree of nicotine inside an agreeable reach.

- Individuals who smoke can immediately get reliant on nicotine and endure physical and enthusiastic (mental or mental) withdrawal manifestations when they quit smoking. These manifestations incorporate crabbiness, anxiety, cerebral pains, and inconvenience dozing. The genuine characteristic of habit, however, is that individuals actually smoke despite the fact that they realize smoking is awful for them - influencing their lives, their wellbeing, and their families' unhealthily. Indeed, a great many people who smoke need to stop.

The following figure shows Arterial and venous levels of nicotine during cigarette smoking.

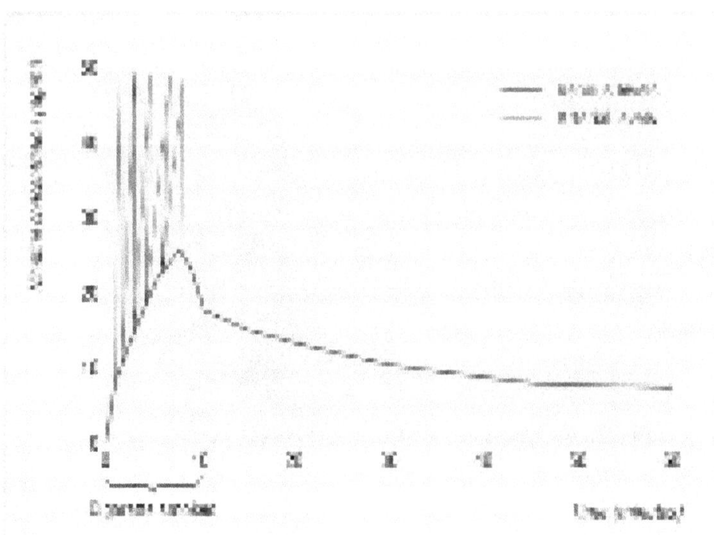

Physical and psychological effects of nicotine

Retention of tobacco smoke from the lung is quick and complete, creating with every inward breath a high focus blood vessel bolus of nicotine that arrives at the cerebrum inside

10-16 seconds, quicker than by intravenous infusion. Nicotine has a distributional half existence of 15-20 minutes and a terminal half-life in blood of two hours. Smokers in this manner experience an example of dreary and transient high blood nicotine focuses from every cigarette, with customary hourly cigarettes expected to keep up raised fixations, and overnight blood levels dropping to near those of non-smokers.

Nicotine slowly affects mind neurochemistry. It enacts nicotinic acetylcholine receptors (nAchRs), which are broadly dispersed in the mind, and instigates the arrival of dopamine in the core accumbency. This impact is equivalent to that delivered by different medications of abuse, (for example, amphetamines and cocaine) and is believed to be a basic element of cerebrum habit instruments.

Nicotine is a psychomotor energizer, and in new clients it speeds basic response time and improves execution on undertakings of supported consideration. Notwithstanding, resistance to large numbers of these impacts before long creates, and constant clients presumably don't keep on getting outright enhancements in execution, psychological handling, or temperament. Smokers commonly report that cigarettes quiet them down when they are focused and assist them with concentrating and work all the more successfully, yet little proof exists that nicotine gives compelling self-prescription to unfriendly disposition states or for adapting to pressure.

The following figure shows the pathways of nicotine reinforcement and addiction.

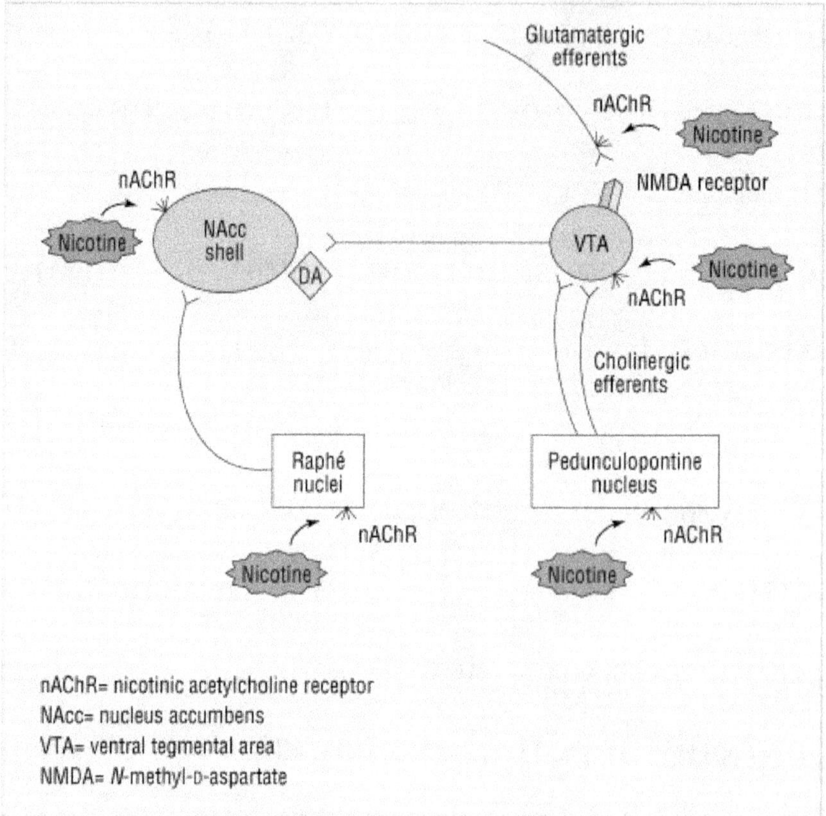

Symptoms of nicotine withdrawal

A significant part of the immovability of cigarette smoking is thought to come from the issues of withdrawal manifestations especially crabbiness, fretfulness, feeling hopeless, impeded fixation, and expanded hunger just as from desires for cigarettes. These withdrawal manifestations start not long after the last cigarette and are at maximal force for the main week. The greater part of the emotional indications at that point resolve more than three or a month, yet craving can endure for a while. Longings, once in a while exceptional, can likewise endure for a long time, particularly whenever set off by situational signals.

Following table shows the effects of nicotine withdrawal.

Symptom	Duration	Incidence (%)
Lightheadedness	< 48 hours	10
Sleep disturbance	< 1 week	25
Poor concentration	< 2 weeks	60
Craving for nicotine	< 2 weeks	70
Irritability or aggression	< 4 weeks	50
Depression	< 4 weeks	60

Restlessness	< 4 weeks	60
Increased appetite	< 10 weeks	70

Regulation of nicotine intake

Smokers show a solid inclination to control their nicotine admissions from cigarettes inside very thin cutoff points. They keep away from admissions that are either excessively low (inciting withdrawal) or excessively high (prompting upsetting impacts of nicotine glut). Inside people, nicotine inclinations arise right off the bat in the smoking vocation and appear to be steady over the long haul. The wonder of nicotine titration is answerable for the disappointment of admissions to decrease in the wake of changing to cigarettes with low tar and nicotine yields. Compensatory puffing and inward breath, working at a psyche level, guarantee that nicotine admissions are kept up.

As nicotine and tar conveyance in smoke are firmly coupled, compensatory smoking similarly keeps up tar admission and annihilations any potential wellbeing acquire from lower tar cigarettes. Comparable compensatory conduct happens in the wake of eliminating the quantity of cigarettes smoked every day; consequently this mainstream technique neglects to convey any important medical advantages.

The figure below shows regulation of nicotine intake; actual and predicted intake per cigarette:

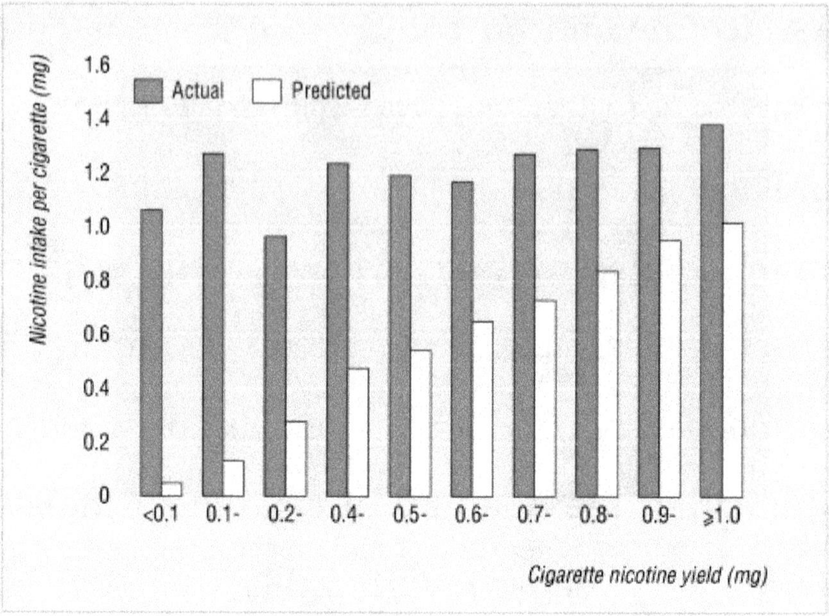

Nicotine intake per cigarette (mg)
1.6
1.4
1.2
1.0
0.8
0.6
0.4
0.2
0
Actual
Predicted
<0.1
0.1-
0.2-
0.4-
0.5-
0.6-
0.7-
0.8-
0.9-
≥1.0
Cigarette nicotine yield (mg)

9+1 Guides to quit smoking

Stopping smoking is probably everything thing we can manage to ensure our bodies from infection, battle sickness, go through therapy, and assist our bodies with mending. Examination shows that 70% of individuals who smoke need to stop and that 41% of smokers have attempted to stop for at any rate one day in the previous year. There are so many reasons why individuals need to stop smoking and better wellbeing is regularly at the first spot on the list. Shockingly, numerous individuals who effectively smoke have had stopped many endeavors that were ineffective; this can be debilitating and it can keep individuals from attempting to stop once more.

It may be very hard to tell how to approach stopping smoking, discover the help you need, what's more, and be fruitful in stopping for great. The substance in this part will give you the key data which you need to see how nicotine reliance happens, what happens when you stop nicotine, how to keep away from the upsetting indications of nicotine withdrawal, and most significantly, how to stop smoking securely and viably.

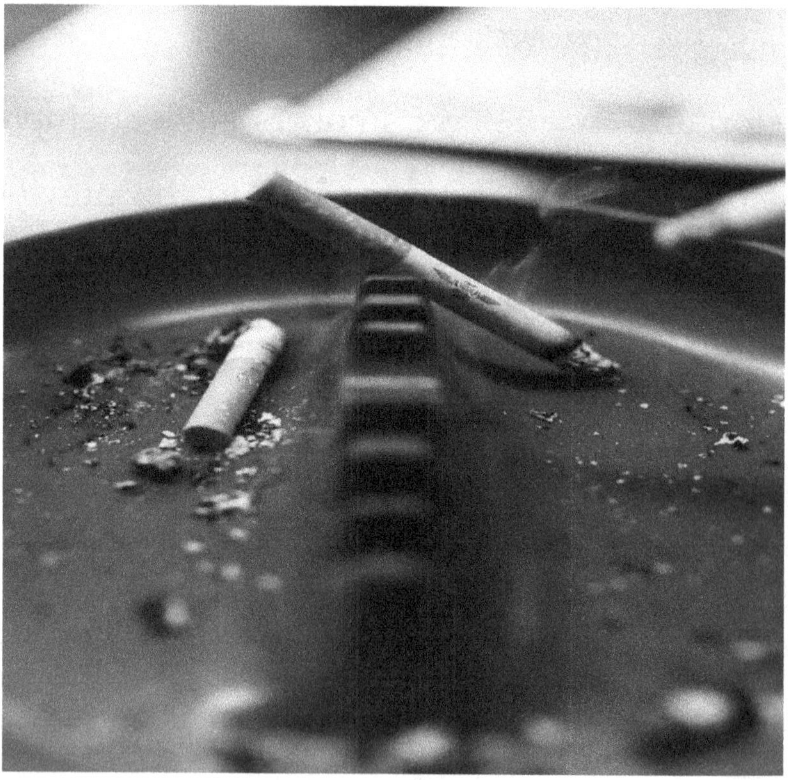

Individuals can stop all alone however it tends to be a test to do this by itself. You will have generally and substantially more achievement in the event that you get backing, advice, and treatment from a medical services proficient or an expert prepared in how to stop smoking. Utilizing nicotine substitution treatment as well as a physician recommended drug to stop in any event duplicates the odds of long haul achievement and at times even quadruples the odds of stopping for great. Following are the ten effective guides to quit smoking:

1. Cutting down to quit

There's no protected degree of cigarette use smoking even a modest quantity can make harm your body. This is the reason there's practically nothing, assuming any, medical advantage from chopping down the quantity of cigarettes you smoke, not at all like stopping completely which has demonstrated medical advantages. Chopping down can, nonetheless, be a decent method to kick you off headed straight toward halting long haul. This is given that you plan well, set the quit date and own it to halting and remaining halted.

While it's in every case best to totally stop smoking on a set date, not every person is prepared to stop straight away. Despite the fact that it's vital to set a quit date inside about a month and a half (shockingly better assuming prior), you can 'slice down to stop' cigarettes over that period, by decreasing the quantity of cigarettes you smoke each day, consistently and fortnight until your quit date.

Well there is some logical proof from enslavement science to back this thought up. Individuals who smoke intensely take in more nicotine and since nicotine is a profoundly addictive substance they will in general need tobacco more and endure all the more sick impacts when they quit utilizing cigarettes. Unmistakably individuals who smoke less cigarettes experience less withdrawal side effects when they attempt to stop. Looking from a less 'clinical' viewpoint, separating an objective that seems unattainable into little reduced down lumps that appear inside your grip frequently is by all accounts a decent procedure.

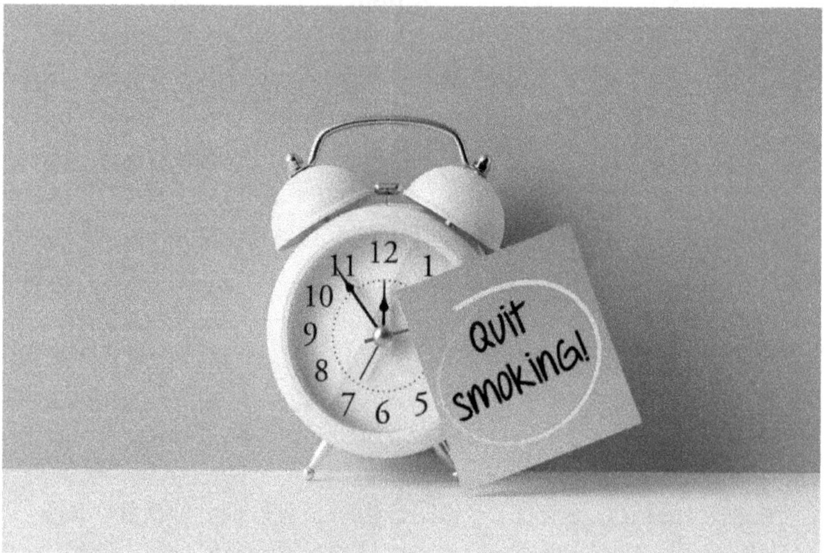

The cutting down to quit method involves reducing your smoking as you move towards a quit date.

It's a bit like taking the slow lane you'll still reach your destination, but the journey might seem a little easier.

Cut down to stop may feel ideal for you in the event that you realize you need to stop smoking, however you're not prepared to stop totally at the present time. By chopping down, you're in any event accomplishing something as you move towards a quit date. Exploration shows that smokers who slice down to stop have a comparative possibility of stopping as the individuals who stop suddenly on their picked quit day. Be that you need to set yourself a quit date prior to beginning to chop down as it may. for this to be successful

The benefit of chopping down to stop is that it permits you to decrease your smoking at your own speed, without squeezing yourself as you move towards your quit date. In case you're thinking about utilizing the slice down to stop technique to quit smoking, we prescribe utilizing these systems to assist you with accomplishing your quit objective:

Work out your 'cut down to stop' time-frame:

- Decide how long you will run after your quit day
- Setting a time span of close to 2 a month to lessen to low levels prior to stopping totally appears to work best.
- Be arranged and prepare:
- Avoid circumstances where you used to smoke
- Take up new exercises to supplant old smoking propensities
- Change the schedules you partner with smoking

- Plan rewards utilizing the cash you save from not smoking
- Get uphold on your stopped smoking excursion:
- Ask your friend help you in your quit endeavor.

Presently you've cut directly down, halting totally is only the following short advance. In the event that you decide to step by step cut down the quantity of cigarettes you smoke every prior day halting by and large, you ought to be cautious that:

- You don't start to compensate for smoking less cigarettes by breathing in more profound and enjoying more drags to get a similar nicotine impact

- Attempting an alternate methodology, for example, cutting down over halting totally, may in the drawn out make it harder for you to stop inside and out.

Once in a while cutting down can be counterproductive and takes more responsibility and order than stopping suddenly. You'll actually encounter a similar withdrawal impacts without seeing the monetary and medical advantages of halting totally. On the off chance that you actually don't feel prepared to stop altogether, you could likewise consider options in contrast to smoking, for example, changing to an e-cigarette what cuts down your danger of damage.

2. Cold turkey

Stopping smoking 'immediately' is the point at which you quit smoking unexpectedly, without utilizing any quit smoking items or expert help.

All you use is your own psychological solidarity to stop and battle desires. This psychological strength is otherwise called 'self-control'.

"Without any weaning period" is a handy solution strategy to stopping tobacco, liquor, or medications. As opposed to continuously tightening the substance, you quit taking it right away.

The term comes from the Goosebumps public once in a while get in the days after they quit, which resemble the skin of a "without any weaning period" in the refrigerator.

A few people go without any weaning period since they figure it will be simpler to quit taking the substance immediately than to tighten. They accept they will not be as enticed to utilize the medication or tobacco item in the event that they simply dispose of it.

Be that as it may, without any weaning period may not be the best method to stop particularly for individuals who are subject to a substance. Stopping excessively fast can prompt awkward withdrawal side effects and a ground-breaking desire to begin utilizing the substance once more.

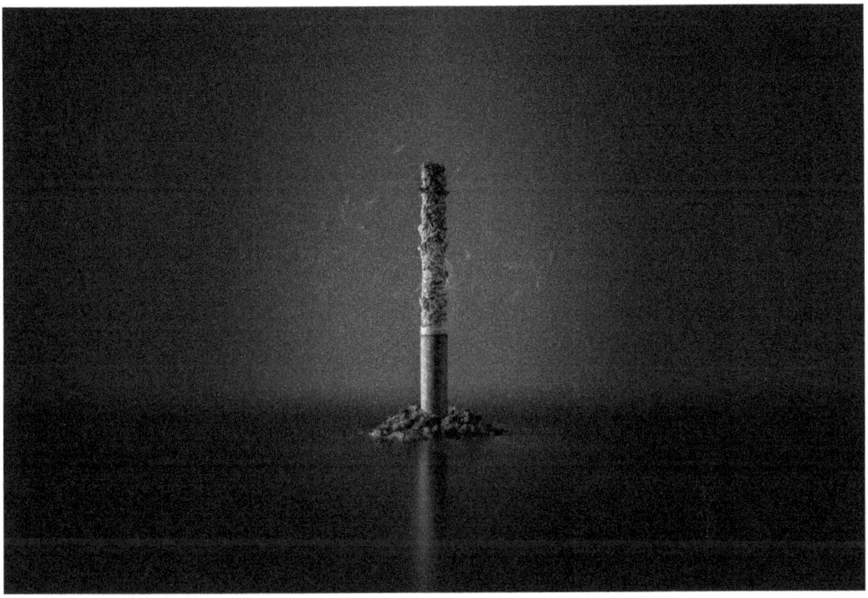

Stopping addictive medications, for example, heroin can be a lot harder immediately. These substances cause actual changes in the cerebrum that lead to serious longings and withdrawal manifestations when you quit taking them.

The security of stopping immediately relies upon the substance you're attempting to stop.

Getting off cigarettes or liquor might be protected to do all alone.

Stopping exceptionally addictive medications or an extreme liquor reliance can cause genuine results, and now and again, demise. It's smarter to be under the consideration of a specialist or compulsion treatment focus.

Your cerebrum gets acquainted with addictive medications, for example, narcotics. At the point when you remove its stock excessively fast, you can create seizures, sporadic heart rhythms, and other withdrawal manifestations. A portion of these manifestations can be not kidding or even hazardous.

Undesirable withdrawal manifestations can drive you back into utilizing the substance again to make them stop. Returning to utilizing a medication or liquor after you've quitted is known as a backslide, after you've stopped, your resistance to the substance is brought down. In the event that you do begin to take it once more, you'll be bound to ingest too much.

At the point when individuals quit smoking 'immediately', they ordinarily build up their own strategies and systems. These might include:

- Setting a quit date or stopping precipitously with no earlier arranging
- Utilizing your own regular mental qualities (self-discipline) to beat desires
- To be fruitful however, 'without any weaning period' stopping will as a rule

require somewhat seriously arranging, for example,

- Evading circumstances where you used to smoke
- Evaluating new exercises to supplant old smoking propensities
- Changing schedules that you partner with smoking
- Bring upheld on your stopped excursion by a companion or relative
- Putting aside the cash you save from not smoking to remunerate yourself later on.

The main activity whenever you've chosen to stop is to call your primary care physician or medical services supplier. A clinical expert can offer you guidance on the most secure approach to stop.

Your PCP can suggest prescriptions and restoration programs that can help. For instance, they can offer physician endorsed medications to facilitate the longings that accompany stopping smoking or narcotic medications.

Additionally, let your loved ones realize that you want to stop. They can help you through the cycle and divert you in case you're enticed to begin utilizing once more.

Dispose of each enticement. On the off chance that you smoke, toss out all cigarettes, lighters, and ashtrays. In the event that you have liquor use issue, spill out the entirety of the liquor in your cooler and wash room. Take any unused prescriptions to a police headquarters or other approved assortment site.

Likewise plan for desires by have heaps of interruptions close by. Bites like carrot sticks and licorice can keep your hands and mouth involved when you need a cigarette. A decent film may take your brain off the desire to utilize drugs.

At last, line up help. Look for help from an expert advisor or specialist. In case you're thinking about stopping smoking 'immediately', it assists with being readied and has systems set up for additional difficult occasions. Here are a few hints and tips:

- Consider your resolve a muscle - the more you use it, the more grounded it gets! In any case, remember that simply like genuine muscles, your self-control muscle can get drained as well…

- In the event that you feel your determination blurring, help yourself to remember the reasons you needed to turn into a non-smoker and recognize how far you've come.
- Or on the other hand, allow your resolution to recuperate by attempting to maintain a strategic distance from basic clearing triggers or testing out another quit strategy.

Have confidence that over the long haul, your resolve muscle will get more grounded, which means it will get simpler to oversee longings and oppose the craving to smoke.

3. Nicotine Gum

Chewing gum is a shockingly antiquated human conduct, going back at any rate 6,000 years. The antiquated Greeks even bit gum with germicide properties to renew their breath! During the 1980s, scientists thought of the astute thought that gum containing nicotine could help individuals quit smoking.

Nicotine gum is a sort of nicotine substitution treatment (NRT) a gathering of items intended to furnish you with a limited quantity of nicotine, without the tar and other destructive synthetic compounds found in cigarettes.

It's a restoratively demonstrated approach to help you quit smoking, by managing the actual side to your nicotine habit. Along these lines, by proceeding to get low degrees of nicotine subsequent to halting smoking, longings and withdrawal side effects are fundamentally diminished, and individuals frequently locate that this makes the stopping cycle significantly less testing. Subsequently, NRT is perhaps the most well-known approaches to stop, and nicotine gums are both normally utilized and generally accessible as stopped smoking guides.

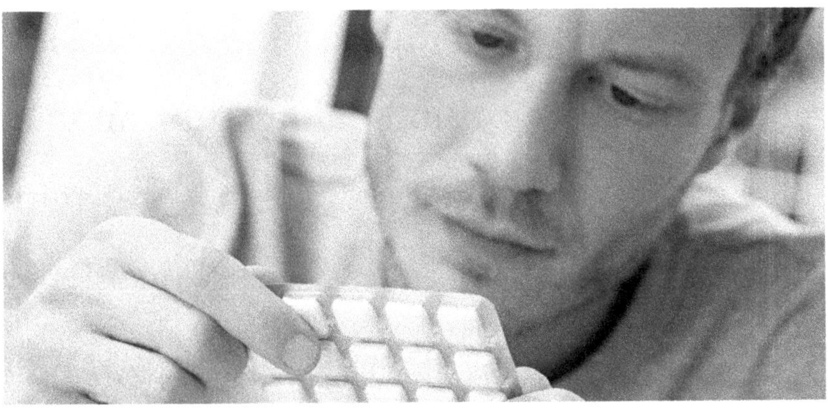

Nicotine gum is an over-the-counter, sedated biting gum that conveys a portion of nicotine orally. It's expected to supplant the nicotine that individuals would somehow or another get from smoking cigarettes or other tobacco items. While it contains the compound liable for the addictiveness of cigarettes, nicotine gum does exclude any of the other frightful substances. It's additionally sans sugar.

It's an experimentally tried item, and exploration shows that it tends to be extremely successful as a quit smoking guide. Nonetheless, it's essential to take note of that the explanations behind taking up smoking and keeping up the propensity are mind boggling, and the dependence on nicotine is just a single contributor to the issue.

Specialists thusly exhort that nicotine gum ought to be utilized related to treatments that focus on the mental components related with smoking, regardless of whether that is through visiting an advisor, or utilizing a proof based virtual treatment like the Quit Genius application. Nicotine gum ought to be utilized related to treatments that focus on the mental factors related with smoking.

If you are attempting to either stop smoking or cut down on the measure of cigarettes you smoke, nicotine gum could help you on your way. While all nicotine substitution treatment items (gums, patches, tablets and so on) are similarly pretty much as successful as one another, you may wish to go with a gum if your yearnings are abrupt, and you require quick help from your manifestations. The demonstration of biting gum itself can likewise be an interruption from smoking, as it can fulfill the oral obsession that regularly results when you surrender cigarettes.

Prior to beginning nicotine gum treatment, you should visit your PCP or address your drug specialist to guarantee that it's appropriate for you, and that you don't have any ailments which could be undermined by utilizing these items. You'll likewise have to advise your PCP or drug specialist regarding any meds you take, including non-remedy items like nutrient enhancements.

It's particularly significant that pregnant ladies or the individuals who are breastfeeding look for clinical counsel prior to utilizing nicotine gum, to check whether utilizing this prescription will have any unfriendly impacts on your child. This likewise applies to ladies who become pregnant during nicotine gum treatment.

Nicotine gums are accessible in two qualities. The particular nicotine portion that you require relies upon the quantity of cigarettes you're accustomed to smoking. When all is said in done be that as it may, on the off chance that you smoke under 25 cigarettes each day, settle on the gums containing 2mg of nicotine and perceive how you get on. In case you're a weighty smoker, you might be in an ideal situation beginning with the 4mg gum.

You should stand by in any event 15 minutes subsequent to eating or drinking prior to utilizing nicotine gum. Like ordinary gum, this item ought to be bitten, despite the fact that there is somewhat of a procedure needed to guarantee a consistent and complete arrival of nicotine. Rehash this cycle until biting no longer delivers the shivering sensation, implying that all the nicotine has been delivered. This can take up to around 30 minutes.

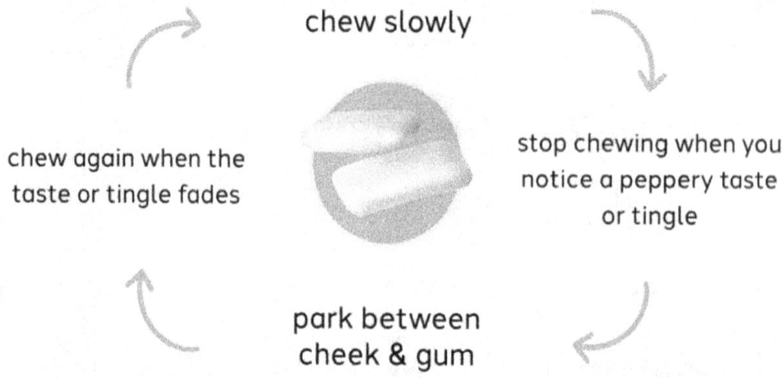

Take care not to swallow the gum and don't bite more than each piece in turn. You can bite up to one piece of gum each hour, so as to decrease the recurrence of utilization as your smoking end program advances. Try not to utilize in excess of 24 pieces in a day.

On the off chance that you miss a portion, don't go through 2 pieces to make for it. Either utilizes a piece of gum when you understand, or basically stand by until the following portion is expected.

Begin utilizing nicotine gum on your quit day, when you'd ordinarily smoke your first cigarette. Nicotine gum is a stopped smoking guide, however it's anything but a drawn out arrangement. Its motivation is to help you battle your habit by making the interaction smoother and simpler to support. While utilizing these items, you're actually conveying an inventory of nicotine into your circulation system, so in the event that you keep on utilizing them uncertainly, you will not have the option to break the actual dependence on nicotine.

All things considered, you'll need to steadily wean yourself off nicotine gum, as both your body and your psyche start to adjust to being without smoke. At the point when you begin utilizing nicotine gum, you should monitor the dates, and work by the accompanying timetable:

- During weeks 1-6: bite 1 piece of gum each 1-2 hours
- During weeks 7-9: bite one piece of gum each 2-4 hours
- During weeks 10-12: bite one piece of gum each 4 to 8 hours

Nicotine gum is a stopped smoking guide, however it's anything but a drawn out arrangement. Nicotine gum isn't intended for delayed use and accordingly shouldn't be utilized for over 12 weeks. On the off chance that you feel that you are as yet battling with nicotine withdrawal indications after the multi week point, look for help from a clinical expert as opposed to proceeding with utilization.

4. Nicotine Lozenge

The nicotine lozenge was presented as an OTC type of nicotine substitution in 2002. It is accessible in 2-mg and 4-mg qualities. The lozenge conveys around 25% more nicotine than the same gum portion. In contrast to the gum, measurement choice depends on the "opportunity to first cigarette" in the wake of waking instead of amount of tobacco use.28 if the primary cigarette is smoked over 1 hour subsequent to waking; the 2-mg structure is a suitable dosing decision. In the event that the principal cigarette is smoked inside 30 minutes of waking, the 4-mg structure ought to be utilized.

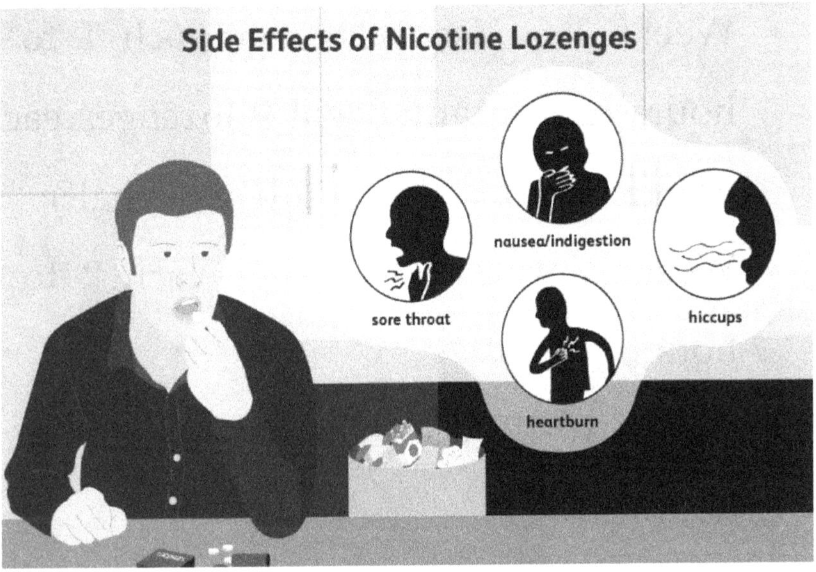

Patients ought to be told not to bite or swallow the lozenge, but rather to move it to various territories of the mouth until it totally breaks down (20 to 30 minutes). Likewise with the gum, utilization of acidic food or drinks 15 minutes prior or during lozenge use will diminish the ingestion of nicotine.

To encourage tightening, urge patients to utilize the lozenge on the accompanying timetable:

- Weeks 1-6: Use 1 lozenge each 1 to 2 hours (use in any event 9 lozenges each day for the initial a month and a half)
- Weeks 7-9: Use 1 lozenge each 2 to 4 hours
- Weeks 10-12: Use 1 lozenge each 4 to 8 hours
- Try not to utilize in excess of 20 lozenges each day

Unintentional swallowing of nicotine can exacerbate active peptic ulcers, and nicotine lozenges should be used with caution in patients with an active history of this disease such as:

- Nausea
- Hiccups
- Cough

- Heartburn
- Headache
- Flatulence
- Insomnia

5. Transdermal Patch Bupropion Sustained Release (SR)

The nicotine transdermal patch is accessible OTC and conveys a consistent portion of nicotine with the most reduced habit capability of all the NRTs. Different transdermal nicotine patch plans are available that fluctuate broadly in detailing, plan, and length of wear (i.e., 16-hour and 24-hour). Plasma nicotine levels got through transdermal conveyance are around half lower than those accomplished with cigarette smoking. Lower levels of nicotine ease the side effects of withdrawal, yet are undeniably more averse to prompt reliance when contrasted and tobacco or different types of NRT.30 Different brands of the transdermal patch have diverse dosing regimens. The clinician should choose the best measurement and routine to address the individual patient's issues. Nicotine patch treatment is utilized to help individuals quit smoking cigarettes. This treatment replaces nicotine in your body that you were getting from cigarettes so you don't have withdrawal indications when you quit smoking.

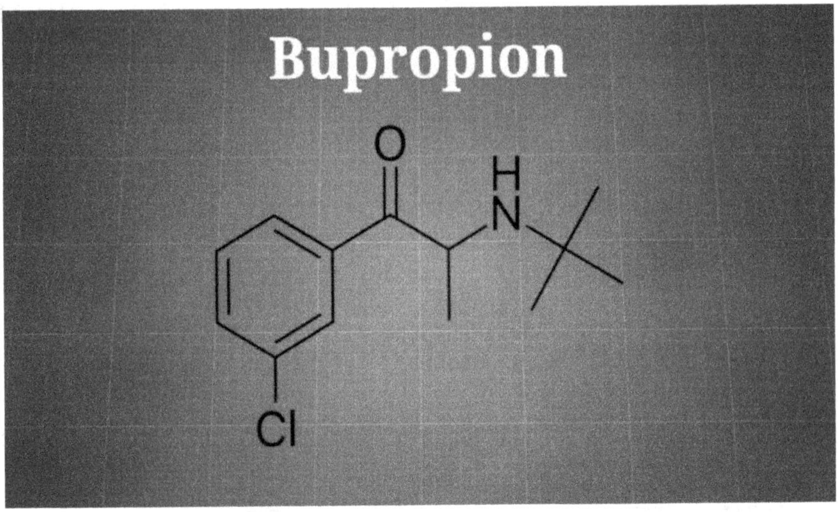

Nicotine patches are applied straightforwardly to the skin. They are applied once every day, as a rule simultaneously every day. Nicotine patches come in different qualities and might be utilized for different periods of time. Follow the bearings on your solution mark cautiously, and ask your essential consideration supplier (PCP) or drug specialist to clarify any part you don't comprehend. Use nicotine skin patches precisely as coordinated. Do not utilize pretty much of them or use them more frequently than endorsed by your PCP.

Prior to utilizing nicotine skin patches, tell your PCP and drug specialist on the off chance that you are oversensitive to sticky tape or any medications. Mention to your PCP and drug specialist what remedy and nonprescription drugs you are taking. Tell your PCP on the off chance that you have or have at any point had a coronary episode, unpredictable pulse, angina, ulcers, uncontrolled hypertension, overactive thyroid, tumor, or a dental condition or turmoil. Tell your PCP in the event that you are pregnant, plan to get pregnant, or are bosom taking care of. In the event that you become pregnant while utilizing nicotine skin patches, call your PCP right away. Nicotine and nicotine skin patches may make hurt the baby.

Albeit results from nicotine skin patches are not normal, they can happen. Tell your PCP if any of these side effects are serious or don't disappear:

- Skin disturbance
- Trouble resting (sleep deprivation)
- tipsiness
- migraine

- furious stomach
- sickness
- regurgitating
- looseness of the bowels
- redness or growing at the patch site

Keep this drug in the holder it came in, firmly shut, and far from youngsters. Store it at room temperature and away from abundance warmth and dampness.

6. Varenicline

Varenicline (trademark Chantix and Champix) is a doctor prescribed medicine used to treat nicotine compulsion. It both lessens needing for and diminishes the pleasurable impacts of cigarettes and other tobacco items. Varenicline causes you quit smoking. To expand your opportunity of accomplishment, utilize this drug with a quit smoking project that incorporates training, backing, and directing. Stopping smoking brings down your danger of heart and lung illness, just as malignant growth. Varenicline works by impeding nicotine's belongings in the cerebrum that make you need to smoke.Discuss the dangers and advantages of this prescription, just as alternate approaches to stop smoking, (for example, nicotine substitution treatment), with your doctor.Varenicline isn't suggested for use by youngsters 16 years or more youthful in light of the fact that it doesn't help this age bunch quit smoking. There are various approaches to utilize varenicline. One path is to marked the calendar to stop smoking prior to starting treatment with this medication. Start taking varenicline as coordinated by your primary care physician, 1 to about fourteen days before the quit date. Take one 0.5-milligram tablet once per day for 3 days, at that point increment to one 0.5-milligram tablet two times every day for 4 days. The portion is gradually expanded to diminish the opportunity of results, (for example, queasiness, irregular dreams). It is alright to smoke during this time. Quit smoking on the quit date. Take the portion recommended by your primary care physician two times every day for the remainder of the treatment time frame (generally 12 weeks).

Another approach to utilize varenicline is to begin taking the medication before you pick a date to stop smoking. Start with the 0.5-milligram tablets and increment the portion as coordinated by your primary care physician. Pick a date to stop smoking that is between days 8 and 35 of treatment. Quit smoking on the date you have picked. Take the portion recommended by your primary care physician for the remainder of the treatment time frame.

In the event that you can't pick a quit date, your primary care physician may guide you to begin taking this medicine and step by step decrease smoking with an objective to stop before the finish of your treatment. Follow your PCP's headings cautiously and decrease smoking as coordinated.

Another approach to utilize varenicline is to begin taking the medication before you pick a date to stop smoking. Start with the 0.5-milligram tablets and increment the portion as coordinated by your primary care physician. Pick a date to stop smoking that is between days 8 and 35 of treatment. Quit smoking on the date you have picked. Take the portion recommended by your primary care physician for the remainder of the treatment time frame.

In the event that you can't pick a quit date, your primary care physician may guide you to begin taking this medicine and step by step decrease smoking with an objective to stop before the finish of your treatment. Follow your PCP's headings cautiously and decrease smoking as coordinated.

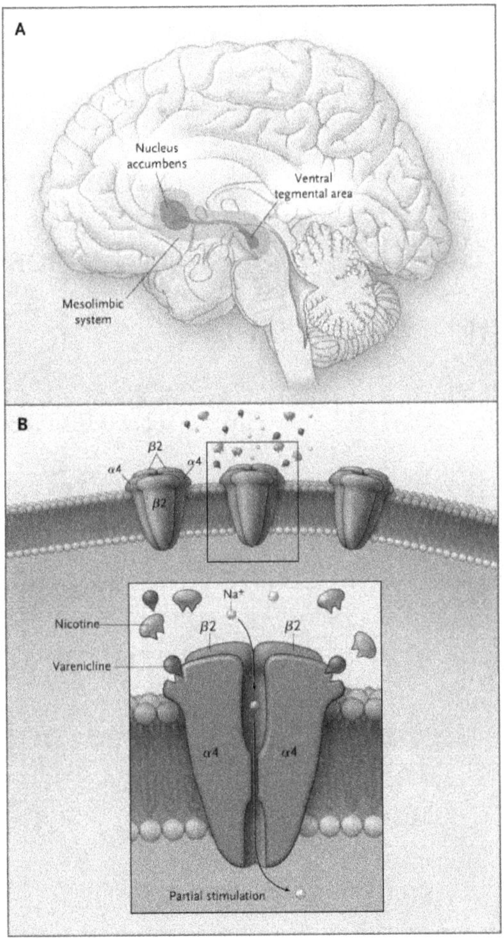

7. Taking non nicotine medications

Most smokers say they need to stop, and around 66% will make an endeavor every year. Notwithstanding, many will decide to make an independent quit endeavor; a technique that has just a little possibility of long haul achievement. The essential motivation behind why numerous smokers think that its hard to stop is a direct result of their reliance on nicotine. Tobacco smoke gives quick conveyance of nicotine to the focal sensory system, where it encourages the arrival of various synapses, for example, dopamine and noradrenaline. In ward smokers, nicotine hardship encourages a withdrawal disorder, comprising of manifestations, for example, fractiousness, low disposition, helpless focus, and inclinations to smoke that can subvert a smokers' endeavor to stop.

Bupropion, an atypical stimulant, is the first, and, up until this point, the solitary non-nicotine treatment authorized for smoking suspension.

There is acceptable reasoning for testing antidepressants for smoking discontinuance, as a solid affiliation exists among smoking and gloom. A higher commonness of smoking exists among individuals who have, or have had a background marked by, despondency. Smokers who are discouraged think that its more hard to stop, a few smokers become discouraged when they quit smoking, and post-end sadness is identified with backslide.

Be that as it may, not all antidepressants have been demonstrated to be useful for smoking end.

Bupropion is ventured to help smokers quit through its capacity to restrain the neuronal reuptake of dopamine and noradrenaline, both significant in nicotine reliance and withdrawal. It might likewise help through its activity as a non-serious inhibitor of the nicotinic acetylcholine receptor, and maybe via its impact on serotonin reuptake. Albeit the exact system by which this drug helps smoking suspension stays questionable, bupropion has been demonstrated to expand forbearance rates and lessen the seriousness of withdrawal indications experienced by smokers when they avoid.

Two crucial result contemplates were distributed in the last part of the 1990s. The originally thought about the impact of three distinctive every day portions (100, 150, and 300 mg) with placebo.24 Results showed a straight impact of an expanding portion on point-pervasiveness discontinuance, albeit no huge contrast was found somewhere in the range of 150 and 300 mg each day at a year follow-up. The subsequent significant examination randomized smokers to get either bupropion (300 mg/day), 21 mg/24 h nicotine fix, both bupropion and fix, or placebo.26 The 1-year constant restraint rates were 18%, 10%, 23%, and 6%, individually. All dynamic medicines were altogether in a way that is better than fake treatment, and bupropion was superior to fix alone. There was no additional favorable position of utilizing a mix routine contrasted and bupropion alone.

Since these examinations, various different investigations looking at the viability of bupropion have been distributed. One Cochrane review10 distinguished a sum of 24 that met their incorporation models. Nineteen investigations, which included in excess of 4000 smokers, taken a gander at the viability of bupropion contrasted and fake treatment. All investigations utilized adjunctive conduct uphold. The meta-investigation showed that, contrasted and fake treatment, bupropion around multiplied long haul restraint rates (OR=2.06; 95% CI: 1.77–2.40).

The viability of bupropion has additionally been analyzed in smokers with smoking-related infection, a populace ordinarily more needy and in this manner harder to treat. Individuals with stable cardiovascular infection treated with bupropion, contrasted and fake treatment, accomplished higher 1-year consistent restraint rates (22% versus 9%).29 When utilized in smokers with gentle to direct COPD, bupropion was related with altogether higher forbearance rates at a half year (16% versus 9%)28 however not at 1 year (10% versus 9%).

Its utilization in forestalling smoking backslide has additionally been inspected. The aftereffects of one examination exploring the utilization of bupropion, contrasted and fake treatment, for a year showed no distinction in persistent forbearance rates between bunches at 1 or 2 years subsequent to stopping.

Another investigation showed no preferred position of utilizing bupropion over fake treatment for forestalling backslide in patients effectively stopping smoking utilizing a nicotine fix. Hence, proof as of now accessible recommends there is little advantage for utilizing bupropion long haul to forestall backslide.

Hardly any examinations have contrasted bupropion and other smoking-end meds. In one of the essential examinations referenced before, bupropion was more powerful than the nicotine fix. Consolidating NRT and bupropion altogether expanded 1-year result contrasted and fix alone (23% versus 10%). Be that as it may, later examinations have not affirmed these outcomes. Further information are required on this issue.

Bupropion is a protected treatment when utilized effectively. Contraindications ought to be checked while recommending this drug. Moreover, a few insurances should be thought of. Smokers with an inclination to seizures ought not take bupropion except if the advantage of smoking discontinuance exceeds any dangers related with utilizing the medicine. Bupropion, in any case, has been discovered protected to use in smokers with stable cardiovascular sickness, without antagonistic impacts on circulatory strain or pulse.

Nortriptyline is a tricyclic upper that restrains the reuptake of noradrenaline and serotonin. It is attempted to act through its noradrenergic system, lessening the seriousness of withdrawal indications. Different theories for its smoking-end properties incorporate its anxiolytic impacts and anticholinergic results, for example, dry mouth, which may make cigarettes less attractive.

The Cochrane survey recognized six randomized-controlled preliminaries that met their consideration measures. These included preliminaries that contrasted nortriptyline and fake treatment just as consolidating nortriptyline and contrasting it and nicotine fix. Out and out, when pooled, the OR was 2.14 (95% CI: 1.49–3.06). Pooling the outcomes from the four investigations that contrasted nortriptyline and fake treatment just, nortriptyline is found to in any event twofold the possibility of long haul forbearance (OR=2.79; 95% CI: 1.70–4.59). An additional favorable position of nortriptyline is that it is a nonexclusive medicine and cheap.

The treatment routine includes a beginning portion of 25 mg/day, expanding progressively over a time of approximately 3 weeks to an objective portion of 75–100 mg/day, which is by and large expected to arrive at a helpful degree of 50–50 ng/ml.The quit date is normally set once restorative levels of the medication have been reached; this may require 10–28 days. The treatment period is ordinarily 12 weeks, with the portion tightened after this. There is restricted proof of advantage for broadening treatment past 3 months.10

The essential worry with utilizing nortriptyline, as other tricyclic antidepressants, is its unfriendly cardiovascular impacts. It is contraindicated in the individuals who have encountered a new myocardial dead tissue or arrhythmias. Extreme liver infection is another contraindication. Also, there are various precautionary measures to note, for example, use in individuals with cardiovascular sickness, a background marked by epilepsy or psychosis, and ladies who are pregnant or breastfeeding.

Nortriptyline has various regular results (for example dry mouth, dazedness, insecurity, and obscured vision). Urinary maintenance, obstruction, sexual troubles, and seizure hazard are likewise announced.

Notwithstanding these, an excess of nortriptyline is ordinarily deadly.

Given that other viable meds for smoking discontinuance are promptly accessible, nortriptyline is presently viewed as a second-line treatment. Besides, it isn't FDA affirmed for smoking end.

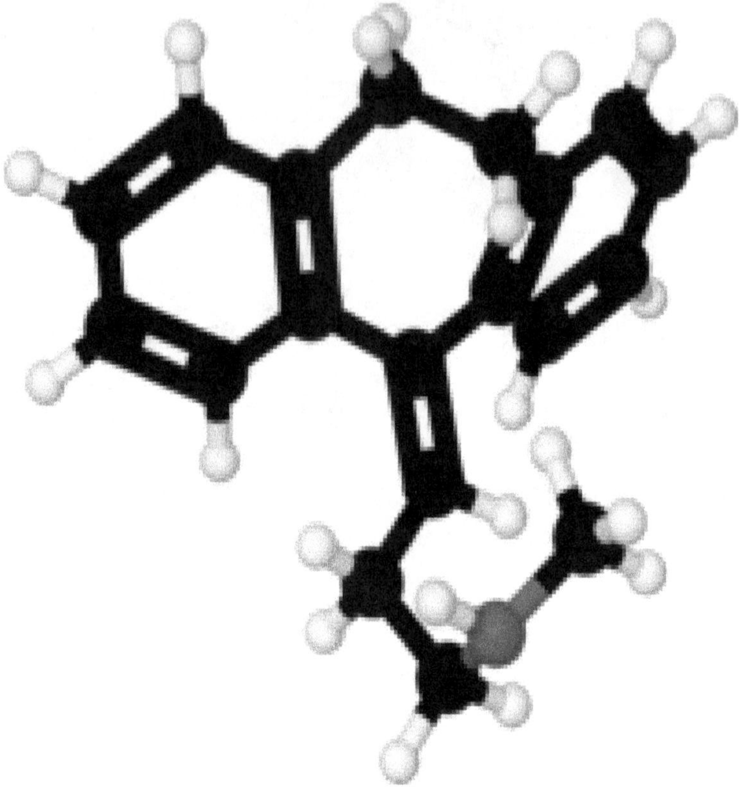

Clonidine has been appeared to improve the manifestations of tobacco withdrawal, and, in certain investigations, increment restraint rates.

The Cochrane survey distinguished a sum of 21 examinations researching its utilization for smoking end. Nonetheless, these were of variable quality, numerous with just present moment follow-up. Just six investigations met the consideration measures, and the pooled results showed an OR of 1.89 (95% CI: 1.30-2.74). This is practically identical with the adequacy of NRT and bupropion Unfortunately, the unfavorable impacts related with this prescription, for example, postural hypotension, unsteadiness and dry mouth, makes its utilization less attractive. Moreover, clonidine causes sedation, albeit this may be of some advantage to the individuals who experience more serious indications of tobacco withdrawal. Gloom, rest aggravation and obstruction are likewise announced, yet these are additionally exemplary indications of nicotine withdrawal, and in this way it is hard to find out which of the two is the causal specialist. Patients with a background marked by sorrow or occlusive fringe vascular infection ought to try not to utilize clonidine.

On the off chance that clonidine is to be utilized for smoking end, at that point treatment ought to be begun 2–3 days prior to stopping, permitting time to arrive at consistent state fixation. It has additionally been utilized in mix with NRT to help oversee withdrawal. Clonidine can be taken orally or through a transdermal fix. Oral portions ordinarily start with 0.1 mg/day, and afterward are slowly expanded, up to 0.4 mg/day. The transdermal portions that have been given are somewhere in the range of 0.1 and 0.3 mg/day. The therapy period is typically short, given over the initial 3 a month subsequent to stopping when withdrawal manifestations are generally serious. After this, the portion is decreased more than a few days, which is especially critical to keep away from hypertensive emergency and hypoglycaemia in individuals with hypertension and diabetes, separately.

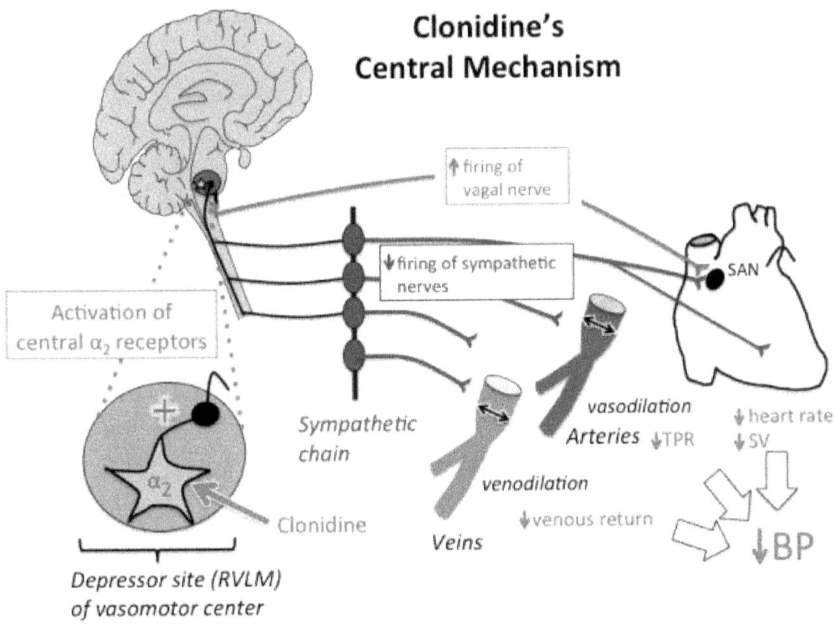

8.Web-based/On-line Support

Existing smoking suspension medicines are tested by low commitment and high backslide rates, proposing the requirement for more inventive, available, and intuitive treatment systems. Twitter is a Web-based stage that permits individuals to speak with one another for the duration of the day utilizing their telephone.

Objective:

This investigation expects to use the online media foundation of Twitter for cultivating shared help to diminish backslide with stopping smoking. Moreover, the examination will look at the impacts of coed versus ladies just gatherings on ladies' prosperity with stopping smoking.

Strategies:

The investigation configuration is a Web-based, three-arm randomized controlled preliminary with two treatment arms (a coed or ladies just Twitter uphold gathering) and a control arm. Members are selected on the web and are randomized to one of the conditions. All members will get two months of blend nicotine substitution treatment (patches in addition to their decision of gum or capsules), sequential messages with connections to Smokefree.gov quit aides, and directions to record their quit date on the web (and to stop smoking on that date) out on the town falling inside seven days of inception of the examination. Members randomized to a treatment arm are set in a completely mechanized Twitter uphold gathering (coed or ladies just), combined with a mate (coordinated on age, sexual orientation, area, and schooling), and urged to speak with the gathering and mate through day by day tweeted conversation subjects and day by day robotized criticism messages (a positive tweet on the off chance that they tweet and an empowering tweet on the off chance that they miss tweeting). Selected online from across the mainland United States, the example comprises of 215 male and 745 female current cigarette smokers needing to stop, matured somewhere in the range of 21 and 59 years. Self-evaluated follow-up reviews are finished online at 1, 3, and a half year after the date they chose to stop smoking, with salivary cotinine approval at 3 and a half year. The essential result is supported biochemically affirmed forbearance at the half year follow-up.

Results: From November 2016 to September 2018, 960 members in 36 gatherings were selected for the randomized controlled preliminary, notwithstanding 20 members in an underlying pilot gathering. Information examination will start soon for the randomized controlled preliminary dependent on information from 896 of the 960 members (93.3%), with 56 members lost to follow-up and 8 dropouts.

Ends:

This examination joins the portable foundation of Twitter with a care group for stopping smoking. Discoveries will illuminate the adequacy regarding virtual distributed care groups for stopping smoking and conceivably clarify sex contrasts in quit rates found in earlier exploration.

Smokers who made quit attempts in the past year

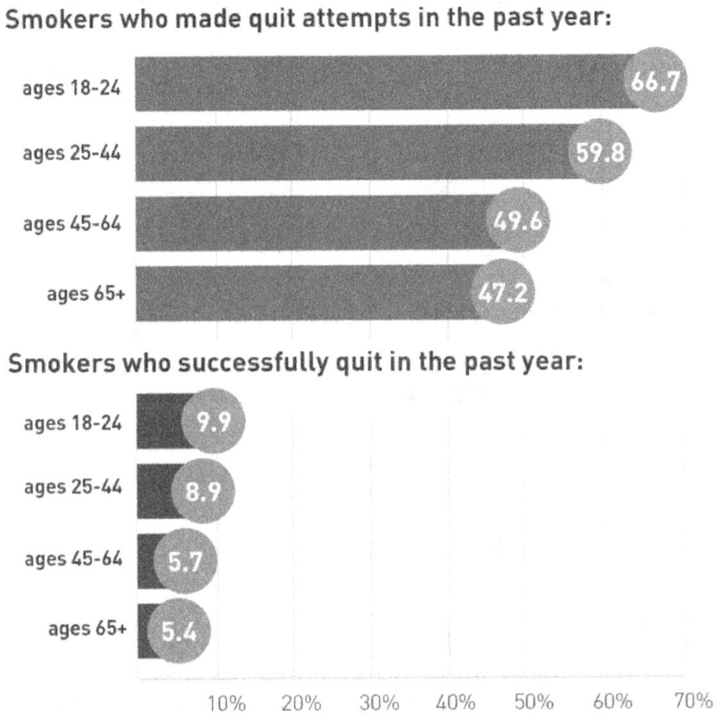

Source: Centers for Disease Control and Prevention, 2017

9. Quit Line

A quitline is a tobacco discontinuance administration accessible through a complementary phone number. Quitlines are staffed by instructors prepared explicitly to help smokers quit. Quitlines convey data, guidance, backing, and references to tobacco clients—paying little heed to their geographic area, race/identity, or monetary status.

Quitlines giving phone guiding to smoking discontinuance get from conduct examination and hypothesis, have been demonstrated to be compelling, and have been received and afterward systematized at both the state and public levels. Despite the fact that analysts have made fundamental commitments to quitline improvement and assessment, this achievement has gone generally unnoticed by the training and exploration networks in clinical, guiding, and wellbeing brain science.

Engineers of a conduct mediation have a fantasy. The substance of their mediation would be gotten from a strong observational and hypothetical establishment. The mediation would be demonstrated to be successful in thorough randomized preliminaries and afterward received by medical care suppliers and frameworks. Following extra corroborative examination, the program would then become systematized, a planned standard help at the nearby, state, or even public level. Scarcely any, conduct programs have accomplished a particularly level of progress. However smoking discontinuance quitlines are moving toward this level.

Quitlines are phone based projects for aiding tobacco clients quit. Tobacco clients start contact with a quitline, and administrations may incorporate sent materials, recorded messages, guiding at the hour of call, callback from an advocate, admittance to suspension drug, or a mix of these administrations. Most administrations are free to the guest.

There are a few favorable circumstances to phone guiding for smoking end. To start with, it is advantageous. Telephone guiding abatements calculated hindrances to treatment and expands administration use. On the off chance that customers need extra assistance over the long run, they can essentially get back to and reconnect in directing. Second, the underlying directing meeting can advance rather rapidly. The semi-mysterious nature of telephone directing encourages genuine conversation, which assists advisors with acquiring an exact clinical picture in a brief timeframe. Third, the phone medium permits guides to give proactive directing (i.e., the instructor calls the customer), in this manner improving the probability that follow-up meetings will happen. Notwithstanding diminishing weakening, proactive advising advances responsibility and social help. Fourth, the phone design fits utilization of an organized directing convention, which gives the base adequate substance to every meeting. An organized convention guarantees that each call is careful yet engaged and brief, making it reasonable for enormous scope application.

Tobacco use is the major, avoidable reason for sickness and passing in the United States, representing 435,000 passings every year . Hence, creating powerful techniques to help tobacco clients quit is in a real sense an immeasurably significant issue. The turn of events and assessment of quitline conventions are an aggregate achievement of numerous specialists, some of them analysts. Albeit the early, original assessment considers were totally distributed in the Journal of Consulting and Clinical Psychology, the vast majority of the resulting work has been distributed in enslavement, clinical, general wellbeing, preventive consideration, or wellbeing training diaries. Theories diaries are not regularly perused by analysts. Quitline intercessions may not be seen as "guiding" or "treatment" by analysts or specialists. Wampold's meaning of psychotherapy is limited to eye to eye cooperations, and California's Board of Psychology doesn't consider phone directing as regulated proficient experience; these hours can't be checked toward licensure. Thus, experts and scientists in clinical, advising, and even wellbeing brain science seem, by all accounts, to be uninformed of quitlines either as an asset for their customers or a chance for their exploration.

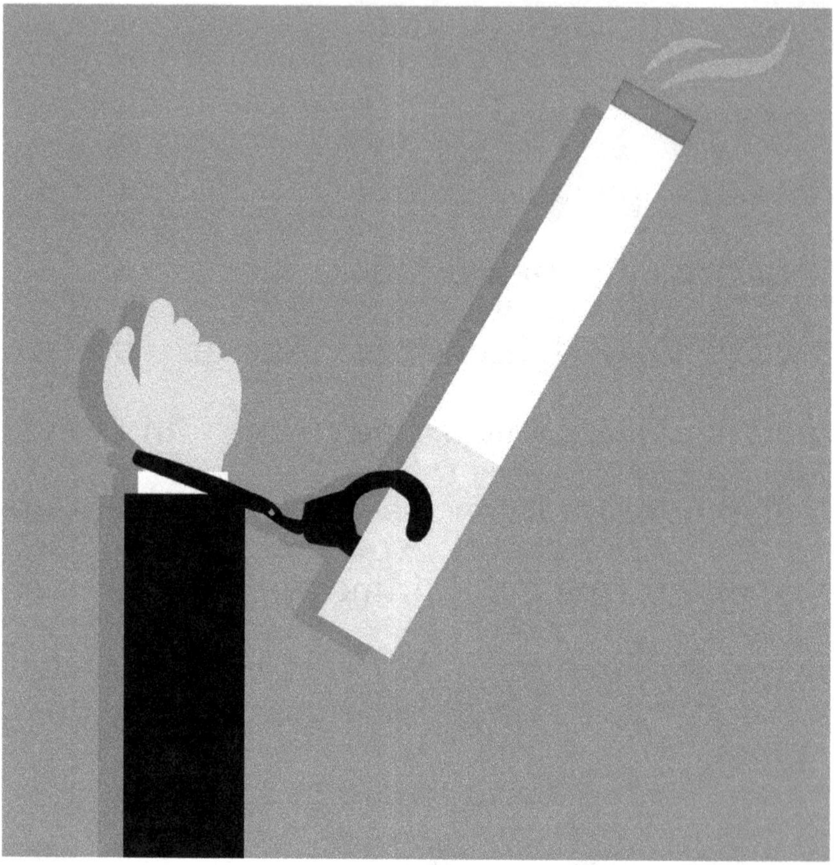

10. Support Groups

Gathering guiding can build your opportunity of stopping by 30%. Individuals are animals of propensity—simply ask a smoker who has attempted to stop. But on the other hand were social creatures, and with regards to stopping smoking, individuals around us can have a major effect. Gathering directing may not be pretty much as successful as some different medicines, (for example, drug), yet for individuals searching for the human touch, it tends to be only the thing.

Quitting through gathering treatment or care groups is to build up an arrangement for putting cigarettes behind you and to master abilities for adapting to yearnings—while collaborating (and shocking tales) with other would-be weaklings. "Steady gathering medicines drove by a talented advocate with others stopping simultaneously are powerful," says Jodi Prochaska, PhD, MPH, a clinical clinician and partner educator at the University of California, San Francisco, who works at the universitys Center for Tobacco Control Research and Education. "Making a guarantee to stop and declaring that obligation to others has been demonstrated to be useful."

Directing and a Nicotine Patch Helped Natasha Quit Smoking

Tobacco use is the major, avoidable reason for ailment and passing in the United States, representing 435,000 passings every year . Hence, creating viable techniques to help tobacco clients quit is in a real sense an incomprehensibly important issue. The turn of events and assessment of quitline conventions are an aggregate achievement of numerous specialists, some of them therapists. Albeit the early, fundamental assessment contemplates were totally distributed in the Journal of Consulting and Clinical Psychology, a large portion of the ensuing work has been distributed in dependence, clinical, general wellbeing, preventive consideration, or wellbeing instruction diaries. Proposals diaries are not normally perused by clinicians. Quitline mediations may not be seen as "advising" or "treatment" by scientists or professionals. Wampold's meaning of psychotherapy is limited to vis-à-vis cooperations, and California's Board of Psychology doesn't consider phone advising as directed proficient experience; these hours can't be checked toward licensure. Subsequently, professionals and analysts in clinical, guiding, and even wellbeing brain science seem, by all accounts, to be ignorant of quitlines either as an asset for their customers or a chance for their exploration.

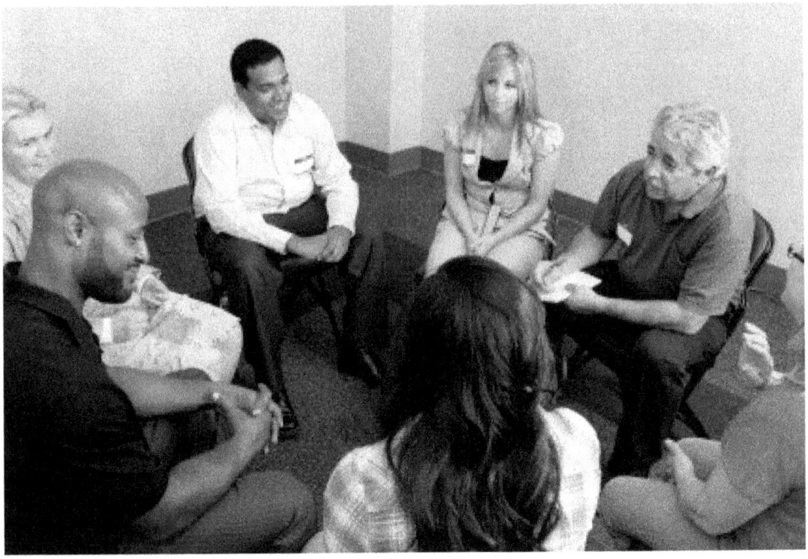

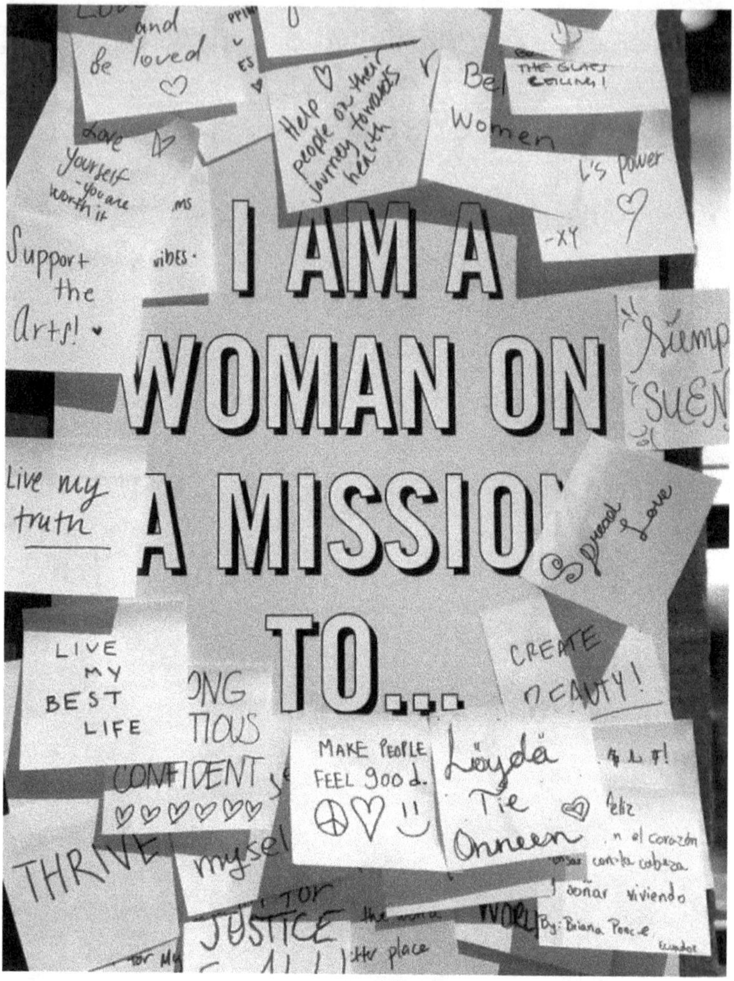

I AM A
WOMAN ON
A MISSIO
TO...
and be loved
Help people on their journey towards health
Women
Love yourself - you are worth it
Support the Arts!
Live my truth
Spread Love
LIVE MY BEST LIFE
CONFIDENT
CREATE
THRIVE
JUSTICE
MAKE PEOPLE FEEL good.
Löydä Tie Onneen
-XY

Prologue

Quitting alcohol is one of the biggest challenges people face. It starts with not knowing you have a drinking problem to accepting it, then gradually working on it while avoiding temptations and situations that put you in that place at the first time along comes staying sober, and finally managing your urges.

One other problem people trying to quit faces is depression. Because alcohol has been their go-to when they are sad or when they want to unwind and take a moment from certain responsibilities, it becomes a challenge and that is when looking for an alternative comes in.

For some people, it is very easy looking for an alternative, either an activity or a non-alcoholic substitute while for others nothing seem to just work. With adequate motivation and zeal, everyone can successfully quit a bad habit.

According to experts, it takes 21 days to quit a habit and they attribute the "21 days to break a habit" myth to Dr Maxwell Maltz, who worked as a plastic surgeon before becoming a psychologist.

In his work, he suggested that it would take about 3 weeks to get used to:

- different facial features after plastic surgery
- the absence of a limb after amputation
- a house they've just moved into

The authenticity of this claim can be questioned as Dr Maltz seemed to rely only on the reports of patients instead of hard scientific evidence. Some persons believe there is a truth in this claim.

In today's world, it has been shown that alcohol use in women increases with each year and the negative effects are far more deleterious in the female gender than their male counterparts. In this book, we will work through a story case study that will help us with practical exercises geared towards enabling you to quit drinking.

"Marie who was born to a not so affluent home grew up becoming very smart lady bagging all the awards from her secondary school days through her University years. She

worked hard and had a passion for the Real Estate Industry and not long after she graduated from the University, a top real estate company offered her a good job. This not only provided her with enough money to take care of her family, but it also expanded her social horizon and by default her lifestyle—attending dinners and Galas and unwinding after work with her colleagues in bars— this spurred new habits. She didn't even notice how these relationships ate deep into her moral fabric. It was safe to say she was a wrecking ball and would soon destroy her standards".

In the next couple of days. We would attempt mechanisms and guides to quit drinking.

What you should know about Alcohol

Alcohol is a psychoactive drug and it is the active ingredient in beer, wine, and spirits. Its recreational activity can be due to the effect on the brain as it causes the release of dopamine— the rewarding hormone—.

Alcoholism which is also known as Alcohol use disorder or excessive alcohol use is a bad drinking habit. It is a medical condition in which a person develops the urge to drink alcohol despite the negative impacts it poses on their lives. The National Institute on Alcohol Abuse and Alcoholism (NIAAA) describes alcohol use disorder as "problem drinking that becomes severe."

What are the different drinking levels?

According to the 2015-2020, Dietary Guidelines for American, moderate drinking can be defined as drinking up to 1 drink per day for women of legal drinking age and up to 2 drinks per day for men of legal drinking age.

When is moderate drinking still too much?

It is safest to avoid alcohol altogether if you are:

- Taking medications that interact with alcohol
- Managing a medical condition that can be made worse by drinking
- Underage
- Planning to drive a vehicle or operate machinery
- Participating in activities that require skill, coordination, and alertness
- Recovering from alcohol use disorder or unable to control the amount they drink
- Pregnant or trying to become pregnant

Excessive alcohol use includes but is not limited to:

- **Binge Drinking**: The term is used to define the heavy consumption of alcohol over a long period. In the United States, the consumption of four or more drinks in a row by women at least once in the previous two weeks can be seen as binge drinking, and the term heavy binge drinking includes three or more such episodes in 2 weeks. Several studies have shown that people who binge drink heavily may have some symptoms of alcoholism.
- **Heavy Drinking**: the National Institute on Alcohol Abuse and Alcoholism (NIAAA) defines heavy alcohol use as more than 3 drinks on a day for a woman

while the Substance Abuse and Mental Health Services Administration (SAMHSA) defines heavy alcohol use as binge drinking on 5 or more days in the past month.

- Any drinking by pregnant women or those under 21

How Long Does Alcohol Stay In The Body?

The mechanism by which alcohol is removed from the body system follows a zero-order kinetic, which means to say independent of the concentration of the alcohol in the system the rate at which it is eliminated from the body is fixed. This is different from the rate of elimination of some other regular drugs where an increase in concentration will also increase the rate at which it leaves the body.

It is on this basis that intoxication occurs. For example; a person that drinks one bottle of 40 per cent alcohol and another that drinks one bottle of 15 per cent alcohol will still eliminate the alcohol within the same duration. With a higher concentration, the risk of increased side effects and toxicity is certain. On average, it takes about 6 hours for a standard drink to be metabolized from the body.

What is a standard drink?

Knowing what counts as a standard drink will help you know the limit of alcohol safe to consume. Many people are surprised to learn what counts as a drink. The amount of liquid in your glass, can, or bottle does not necessarily match up to how much alcohol is actually in your drink. Different types of beer, wine, or malt liquor can have very different amounts of alcohol content. For example, many light beers have almost as much alcohol as regular beer - about 85% as much. Here's another way to put it:

- Regular beer: 5% alcohol content
- Some light beers: 4.2% alcohol content

How do you know how much alcohol is in your drink?

It is important to know how much alcohol your drink contains. In the United States, one "standard" drink (or one alcoholic drink equivalent) contains roughly 14 grams of pure alcohol, which is found in 12 ounces of regular beer, which is usually about 5% alcohol, 5 ounces of wine, which is typically about 12% alcohol, 1.5 ounces of distilled spirits, which is about 40% alcohol.

Even though they come in different sizes, the drinks below are each example of one standard drink.

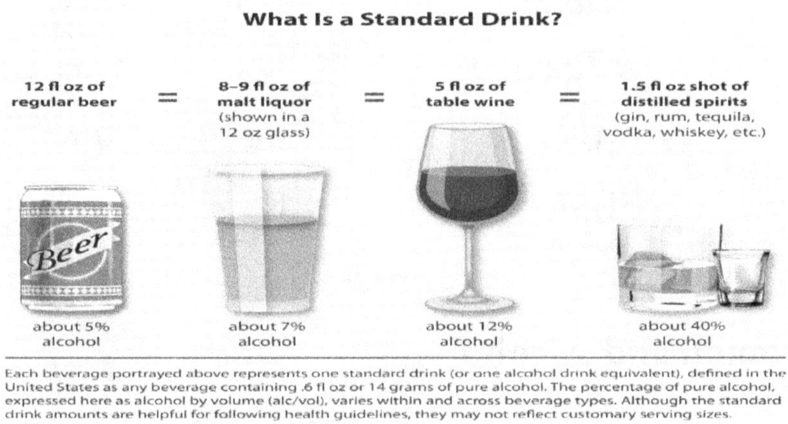

** The above image was extracted from the NIAAA website*

Below is a table with the definition of a standard drink based on different countries.

One Standard Drink by Country

(grams and milliliters of alcohol)

Australia	10 g	13 mL
Canada	13.6 g	17 mL
Ireland	10 g	13 mL
New Zealand	10 g	13 mL
UK	8 g	10 mL
USA	14 g	18 mL

Women and Alcohol

A survey done on the 21 of August 2019 among young youths in the US showed that about 32% of female high school students consumed alcohol compared with 26% of male high school students. Binge drinking was also more common among female (15%) than male (13%) high school students. A 2020 report published in the American Journal of Preventive Medicine found that both current alcohol use and binge drinking among pregnant women aged 18–44 years in the United States increased slightly from 2011 to 2018, both for current drinkers (those having at least one drink of any alcoholic beverage in the past 30 days) and Binge drinkers. Alcohol affects women more different than their male counterparts. The reason for this claim can be attributed to body structure and chemistry. The body of a woman contains less amount of water and more fat cells (adipose) as opposed to the male body which has lesser fat cells. Water dilutes alcohol resulting in lower concentrations in the system and fat retains/stores alcohol exposing the organs to higher. concentrations. So for women, the latter is the case as they possess more fat cells. Another reason for this claim is the reduced quantity of the enzymes alcohol dehydrogenase. This enzyme is responsible for the breakdown of alcohol before it gets to the bloodstream. So at any given amount, the blood level of alcohol will be higher in females than in males and so are the negative consequences.

Seeing the figures of alcoholism rise every year coupled with the more deleterious effect it has on the female gender, for the next four weeks we are going to follow a step-by-step guide in quitting this bad drinking habit.

START WITH A DECISION.

WEEK ONE

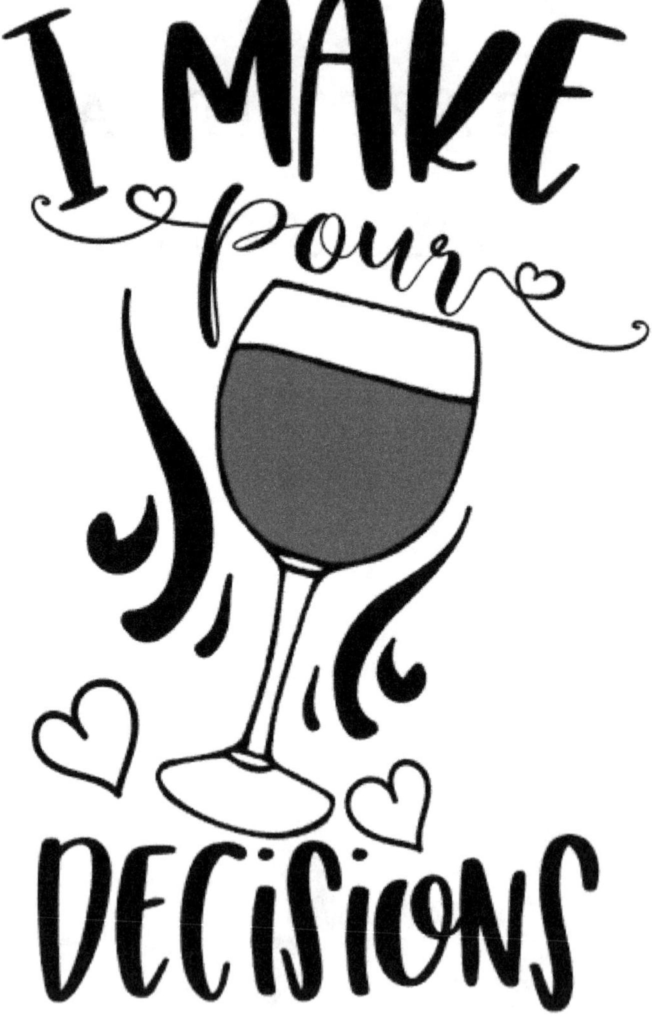

Day ONE

Not knowing when it is a Problem

"Marie has had a terrible day at work, apparently she wasn't prepared for her big pitch to secure the multimillion naira contract for her company. After elevating to the position of the Assistant Manager at her company, she relaxed and got very complacent. On the day before her big presentation that was expected to close a huge deal, she was out with the girls. She has had a history of a drinking problem although it wasn't diagnosed yet. One too many times she ended up drinking more or longer than she intends and this night was one of those nights.

She was out clubbing with Sophie and Claire and had consumed much more than she had ever consumed. The last time it happened, she had woken up from bed to a total stranger beside her in her house and she had no idea how she got home from the bar. She always promised herself after several recurrences that she would stop, she always ended up feeling depressed after the deed had been done.

On this fateful evening, Marie just wanted to ease off the anxiousness and tension about her "big day" so she opted for going to the karaoke with Claire and Sophie. They got into a game that involved a penalty of drinking booze if you couldn't complete the lyrics of a song. She just wanted to ease the tension and she delved into the game, she kept on losing and consequently drinking. She was surprised at how much she had consumed without flinching. They teased her saying she drank like a fish. It was all fun and games until one of the guys invited her and her friends to a club nearby.

—The next morning—

Marie woke up not knowing where she was but was grateful she still had her sanity. Not knowing where she was and how she got there, she reached out to get her phone and it was dead. She looked at her watch lying in one corner of the room and jumped up when she saw the time. It was 9:30 am and her presentation was for 9:00 am making her 30 minutes behind schedule.

At 11:00 am Marie was at her workplace. She rushed into the conference room that showed all forms of tardiness. She started setting up for her presentation and asides from her tardiness, she was in utter confusion mixing up her slides and sounding very incompetent. The Presentation lasted for a very short 15 minutes and her supervisor had never been more disappointed with a project as she was with Marie's. She was the brightest and youngest staff and he would have placed a bet on her nailing this presentation. But now he wouldn't talk to her, and she was frustrated. He sent her a message later saying he will contact her after a decision has been made.

Marie got back home feeling very depressed and sad, to say the least. Until now she hasn't admitted that she has a drinking disorder. All these wouldn't have happened if she had not taken any drink or partied that night, her friends were at her house. They explained they were also wasted from the alcohol at the game that they didn't notice her leaving. By this time they already aware of her awful presentation. She sat on her couch, still on her work clothe with five empty bottles of alcohol and a half-empty bottle of beer in one hand. Claire attempted to stop her from drinking but she fought back so she dragged the bottle of beer from her".

It only takes a few mild symptoms to signal the beginning of a drinking problem, knowing these disturbing signs, and working on them on time can help prevent a drinking disorder. Carefully look at the exercise below, do you see any familiar symptoms in yourself? If Yes, don't worry this 28 days step by step guide will help reduce your risks.

- ***Exercise***

In the past year (tick all that applies), have you:

  - *Had times when you ended up drinking* ***more, or longer,*** *than you intended?*
  - *More than once wanted to* ***cut down or stop*** *drinking, or tried to, but couldn't?*
  - *More than once gotten into situations while or after drinking that* ***increased your chances of getting hurt*** *(such as driving, swimming, using machinery, walking in dangerous areas, or having unsafe sex)?*
  - *Had to drink* ***much more*** *than you once did to* ***get the effect*** *you want? Or found that your* ***usual number*** *of*

*drinks had **much less effect** than before?*

- *Continued to drink even though it was making you feel **depressed or anxious** or adding to another health problem? Or after having had a **memory blackout?***
- *Spend a **lot of time** drinking? Or being sick or getting over other after-effects?*
- *Continued to drink even though it was causing **trouble** with your **family** or **friends?***
- *Found that drinking- or being sick from drinking- often **interfered with taking care** of your **home or family**? Or caused job troubles? Or **school** problems?*

- *o* ***Given up*** *or* ***cut back*** *on* ***activities*** *that were important or interesting to you, or gave you pleasure, to drink?*
- *o More than once gotten* ***arrested,*** *been held at a police station, or had other* ***legal problems*** *because of your drinking?*
- *o Found that when the effects of alcohol are wearing off, you had withdrawal symptoms such as trouble sleeping, shakiness, restlessness, nausea, sweating, a racing heart, or a seizure? Or sensed things that were not there (hallucination)?*

***The questions listed above are based on symptoms for alcohol use disorder in the American Psychiatric Association's**

Diagnostics and Statistical Manual (DSM) of Mental Disorders, Fourth Edition.

The symptoms at the beginning of the list indicate less severity, but as we go down the list, there is likely to be major concerns as she experiences on or more of the symptoms down the list.

Following Marie's story, we can tick five of these symptoms with one or two of the symptoms appearing towards the end of the list raising a cause for concern. Now it's your turn.

Am I?

LOVE

I Am!

Day TWO

Make a list of pros and cons

Recovery for people with a drinking habit as with any other habit is a gradual process. In the early stages, most people are faced with denial. In the case of Marie, it had to take putting her job on the line to realize that she might have a drinking problem. Sometimes even after acceptance, you might find yourself making excuses and dragging your feet. If you find yourself in this position where you are struggling with the decision. Knowing the benefits and the costs of each choice has been proven to help people with their ambivalence about quitting drinking.

Evaluating the Pros and Cons of drinking

In today's exercise, you will be making a table similar to what is below weighing the Pros and Cons of not drinking to the Pros and Cons of drinking but before you start this exercise practice first by making a list of Pros and Cons from the case study "Marie" above. Have fun doing that and see you tomorrow.

Exercise:

Drinking	*Not Drinking*
Is drinking worth the cost?	
Pros	*Pros*
• *It helps me forget about my problems.* • *I have fun when I drink.* • *It is my way of relaxing after a stressful day.*	• *My relationship would probably improve.* • *I'd feel better mentally and physically.* • *I'd have more time and energy for the people and activities I care*

	about.
Cons	*Cons*
• ***It causes problems in my relationship.***	• *I'd have to find another way to deal with problems.*
• ***I feel depressed anxious and ashamed of myself.***	• ***I'd lose my drinking buddies***
• ***It gets in the way of my job performance and family responsibilities.***	• ***I'd have to face the responsibilities I've been ignoring.***

Day THREE

To Cut Down Or To Quit

The decision to quit or cut down on your drinking problem will depend on the severity of the problem. If you're an alcoholic—which, by definition, means you aren't able to control your drinking—it's best to try to stop drinking entirely. But if you're not ready to take that step, or if you don't have an alcohol abuse problem but want to cut back for personal or health reasons, the following tips can help:

- Set your drinking goal: There is an entire exercise on setting your goals and following through in the next chapter (Check Day Four).
- Choose a limit for how much you'll drink, but make sure your limit is not

more than one drink a day as a woman and try to have some days each week when you won't drink alcohol at all.

- Write your drinking goal down and keep it where you will frequently see it, such as on your phone or taped to your refrigerator. Check Day four.
- Cut down drinking at home: Eliminate or limit the quantity of alcohol you keep at home. It's much easier to avoid drinking if you don't keep temptations around.
- Drink slower: When you drink, sip slowly and take a break of 30 minutes or one hour between drinks. You can also switch to drinking soda, water, or juice but not alcoholic drinks.

- Drinking on an empty stomach is always a bad idea, so make sure you drink on a full stomach.

Practice:

Schedule one or two alcohol-free days each week. Then, try to stop drinking for one week. Get a Journal and make a note in it about how you feel physically and mentally these days—recognizing the benefits may help you to cut down for good.

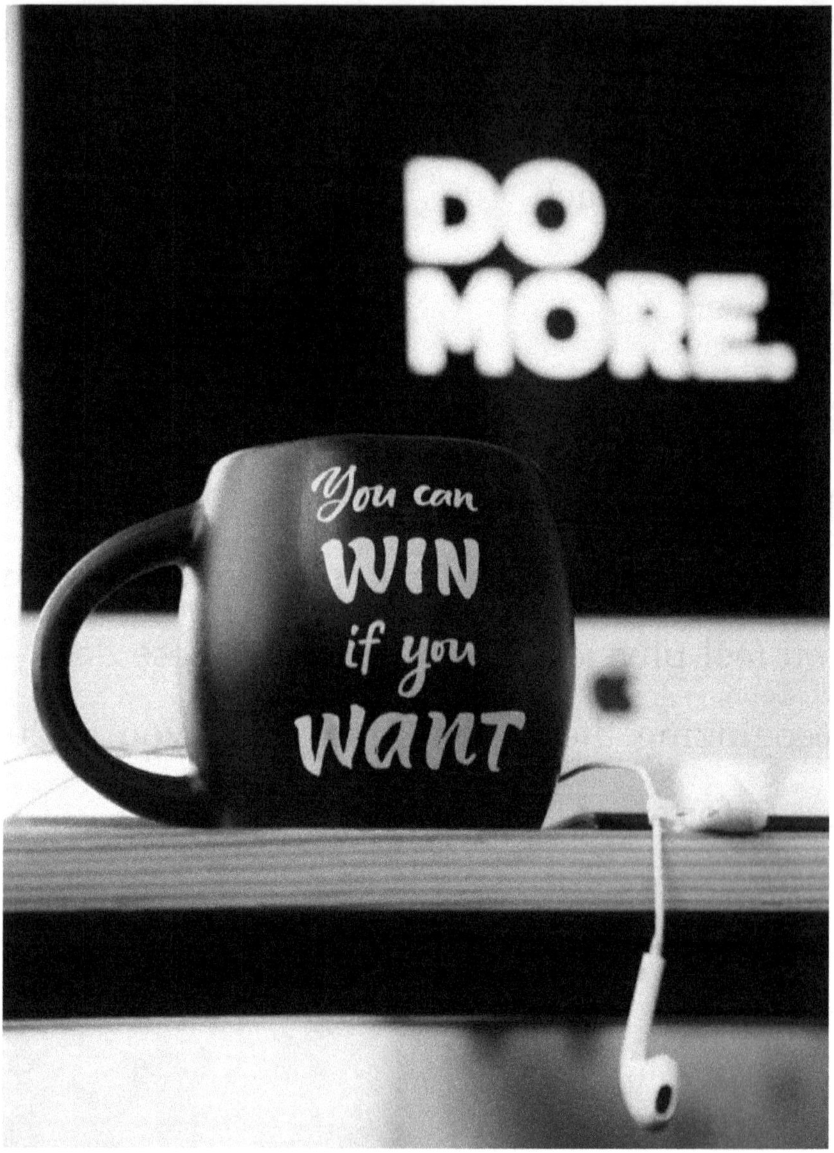
DO MORE.
You can WIN if you WANT

Day FOUR

Set A Goal

Set goals and prepare for change. Once you've decided to change, the next step is establishing clear drinking goals.

The more specific, realistic, and clear your goals are, the better.

Example #1: My drinking goal

I will stop drinking alcohol. My quit date is __________.

Example #2: My drinking goal

I will stop drinking on weekdays, starting as of __________.

I will limit my Saturday and Sunday drinking to no more than three drinks per day or five drinks per weekend. After three months, I will cut back my weekend drinking even more to a maximum of two drinks per day and three drinks per weekend.

Do you want to stop drinking altogether or just cut back?

If your goal is to reduce your drinking, decide which days you will drink alcohol and how many drinks you will allow yourself per day as shown in the latter part of the examples above. Try to commit to at least two days each week when you won't drink at all.

For those completely cutting done, when do you want to stop drinking or start drinking less? Tomorrow? In a week? Next month? Within six months?

If you're trying to stop drinking, we are set a specific quit date.

Practice:

Set a specific quit date on your journal (it must be easily accessible).

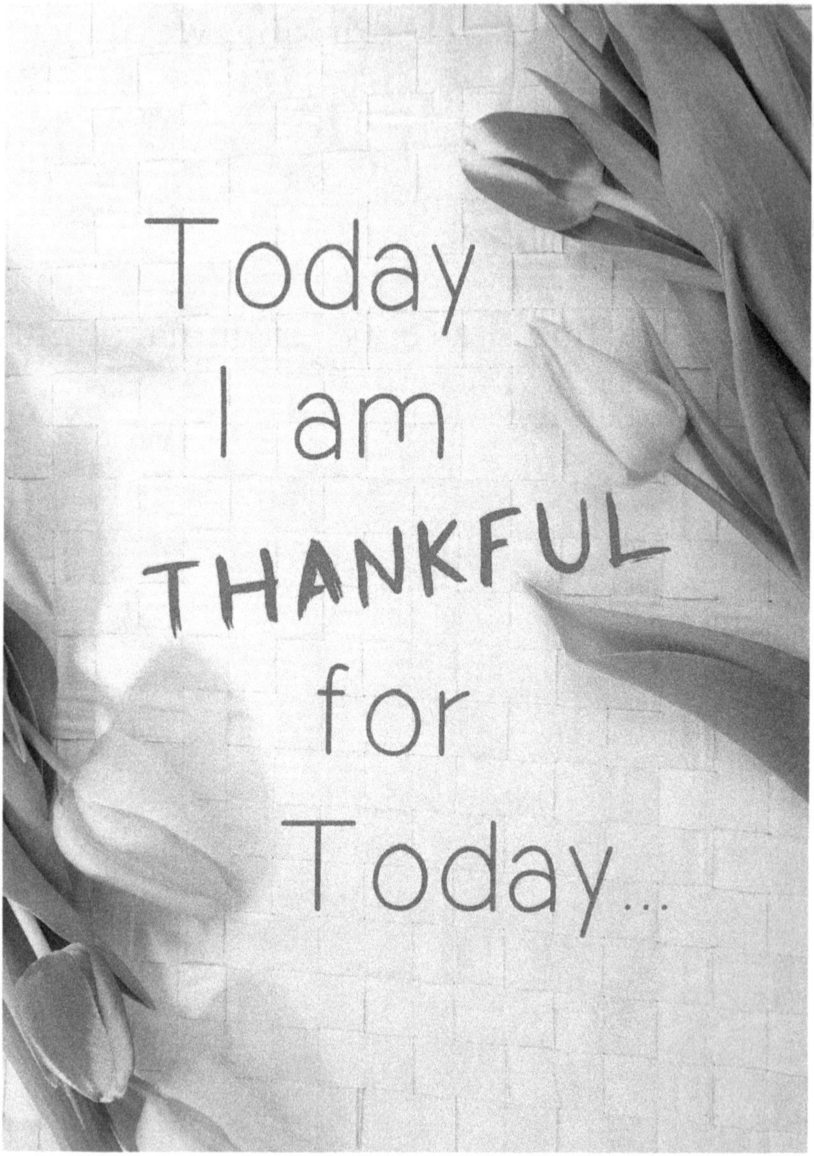
Today
I am
THANKFUL
for
Today...

Day FIVE

Accomplish Your Goals

After you've set your goals to cut back on your drinking, write down some ideas on how you can help yourself accomplish these goals.

For example:

Get rid of temptations: Remove all alcohol, barware, and other alcohol-related paraphernalia from your home and office.

Announce your goal: Inform your friends, family members, and co-workers, let them know that you're trying to stop or cut back on drinking. If they drink, ask them to support your recovery by not doing so in front of you.

Be upfront about your new limits: Make it clear that drinking will not be allowed in your home and that you may not be able to attend events where alcohol is being served.

Avoid bad influences: You may end up losing friends and social connections, but not to worry, the right one will come. Once you have set up these limits. Separate yourself from people who don't support your efforts to stop drinking or respect the limits you've set. This may mean giving up certain friends and social connections, but not to worry, you'll get more.

Experience is the best teacher: Reflect on previous attempts to stop or reduce your drinking.

What worked? What didn't? What can you do differently this time to avoid pitfalls?

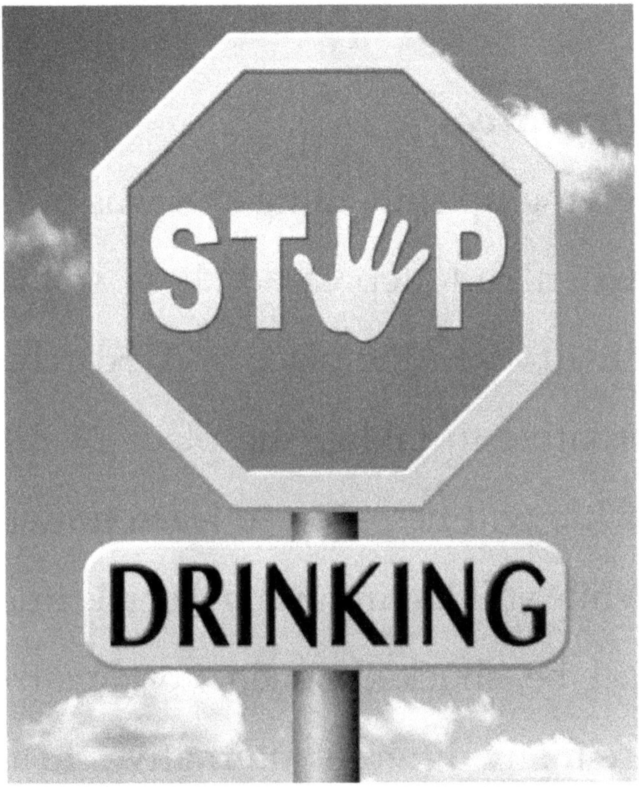
STOP
DRINKING

Day Six

Find alternatives

When giving up something that was once your go-to when sad depressed. It is safe to get something to take the place of it. Searching for an alternative to taking the place of drinking in your life will help you to learn how to stay sober while still having fun in social situations. You will be shocked when you realize that there are many different alternatives to alcohol that people turn to in social gatherings to have the satisfaction that makes them feel as though they are drinking without actually risking their sobriety. Have in mind that even a small amount of alcohol can trigger uncontrollable urges if you are a recovering alcoholic.

These alternatives are meant to help you to feel good and achieve muscle relaxation without exposing you to alcohol capable of causing you an addiction or drinking problem. Below is an outline of suggested alternatives to alcohol gotten from the website of the National Institute on Alcohol Abuse and Alcoholism (NIAAA). Be sure to practice these tips with a sober buddy, sponsor, or mentor to help you achieve your long-term recovery goals.

Here are some of the best alternatives to alcohol consumption:

Alcohol-free drinks (Non-alcoholic beverages)

Try non-alcoholic beverages/beer instead of risking any amount of alcohol consumption. You will get the taste of beer and have something to hold in your hand in social situations where the people around you are drinking. There are even alcohol-free mixed drinks ("mocktails") that taste the same without the negative effects of alcohol.

Additionally, drinks that are carbonated, sparkling, or have a tang to them, such as kombucha, can make you feel like you are drinking alcohol, even though you are completely sober. And the even bigger, long-term benefit of this is that it is better for your physical and mental health.

However, you should note that alcohol-free beers and mocktails do not help everyone. If you are already in recovery and do not have much sober time, these imitation drinks could hinder rather than help your sobriety.

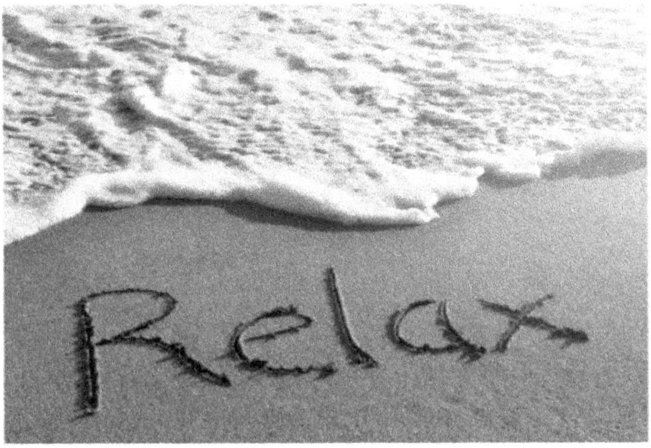

Take time for yourself...

Try muscle relaxation techniques

So many people turn to alcohol to find that sense of relaxation. However, using alcohol to relax does not get to the root problem of why you are experiencing stress in the first place. Guided meditation, exercise, progressive muscle relaxation, yoga, deep breathing, and massage are all alternatives to the release you might feel when you initially pick up a drink.

Set up friend hangouts in places without alcohol

Sometimes, meeting friends at a bar is just not what's best for your recovery needs. Every so often, suggest an alternative plan to hang out—whether that's going on a hike, park, bowling, seeing a movie, etc., you can still find ways to have fun with your loved ones without

the glaring temptation of alcohol.

Day Seven

Reminder strategies

Breaking a habit may be difficult at the initial stage, that is why it helps to have concrete reminders of why and how you've decided to do it. Some standard options include carrying a change plan (More details in Week two) in your wallet or posting sticky notes at home.

Also, consider these high-tech ideas:

Fill out a change plan (refer to week two), email it to your personal (non-work) account, store it in a private online folder, and review it weekly.

Store your goals, reasons, or strategies in your mobile phone as short text messages or notepad entries that you can retrieve when an urge hits.

Set up an automated mobile phone or email calendar alerts that deliver reminders when you choose, such as a few hours before you usually go out. (Email providers such as Gmail and Yahoo mail have online calendars with alert options.)

Create passwords that are motivating phrases in code, which you'll reinforce each time you log in, such as Poco-a-poco, No pain no glory. etc.

Exercise:

Write down Ten (10) motivational phrases or Puns.

WEEK TWO

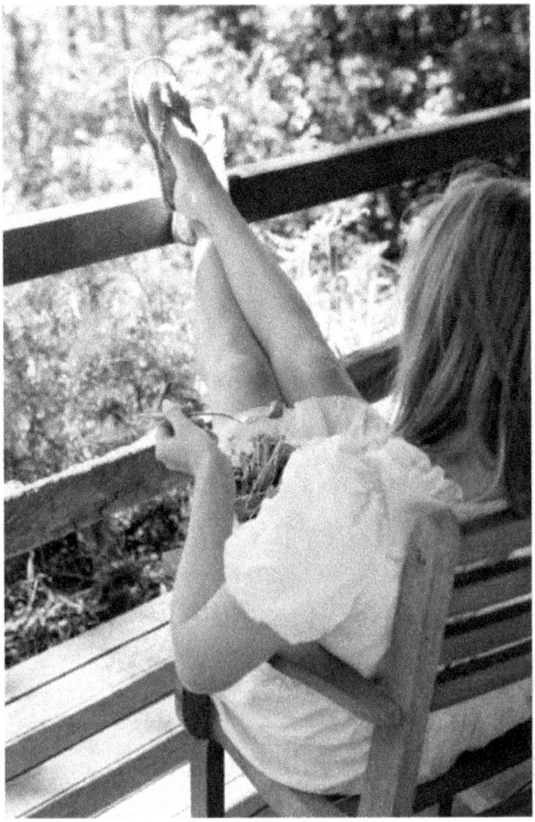

All of Marie's life, she always dreamt of being in a position where she could be able to provide decent and affordable housing for the low-income earners. Growing up in a shanty neighbourhood with moribund buildings and waking up each day thanking God the roofs didn't fall on you while you

were asleep drove her into studying real estate and management. So you can imagine how disappointed and depressed she was after her horrible presentation that would have secured a contract capable of changing the lives of many.

Marie was so good at her job, her follow up on the project was more than anyone could offer. After much consideration, she was awarded the contract and was still placed on four-month probation where she had to attend compulsory Alcoholics Anonymous AA meetings and submit attendance and progress sheets to her company.

This was enough motivation for her and she religiously attended her meetings.

Before we start this week, let us try to identify our motivation, we will be required to go back to this from time to time so I advise you to write it somewhere that is very accessible.

DAY EIGHT AND NINE

Keep Drinking Track

If you want to cut back or quit your drinking, start by keeping track of *every* drink. Find what works best for you. It can also help if you carry a drinking tracker card in your wallet, make check marks on a kitchen calendar, or enter notes in a mobile phone notepad or personal digital assistant.

Making note of each drink before you drink it may help you slow down when needed.

Below are two different forms (Drink tracking cards) you can print, cut out, and keep with you. Both of them help make you aware of patterns and are a key step in planning for a change. Try one form, or try both to see which is more helpful.

The **4-week tracker card** is a simple calendar form. If you mark down each drink before you have it, this can help you slow down if needed.

GOAL: No more than_____drink(s) on any day and _____per week.

Sun	Mon	Tue	Wed	Thu	Fri	Sat
1	2	3	4	5	6	7

Total=

Sun	Mon	Tue	Wed	Thu	Fri	Sat
8	9	10	11	12	13	14

Total=

15	16	17	18	19	20	21

Total=

22	23	24	25	26	27	28

Total=

Date	Situation (People, place, activities) or Triggers (Incidents, feelings)	Type of drink(s)	Amount	Consequences

***Alcohol Analyzer card extracted from NIAA: This will help to note people, places that**

trigger the feelings or urges, the type of drinks offered by the person or in that gathering, the amount and the consequences after consumption which are all useful tools when to prevent recurrences.

Day Ten and Eleven

Count and measure

We have talked about what a standard drink is, knowing the standard drink sizes so you can count your drinks accurately is very useful for individuals who want to cut down on their drinking, So if you skipped the prologue, this is the best time to go back and understand what a standard drink is.

The next step is to measure drinks at home. Away from home, it can be hard to keep track, especially with mixed drinks, and at times, you may be getting more alcohol than you think. With wine, you may need to ask the host or server not to "top off" a partially filled glass.

Kindly turn over to get a list of some drinks and their alcohol content.

Stay Safe and Know your Limit

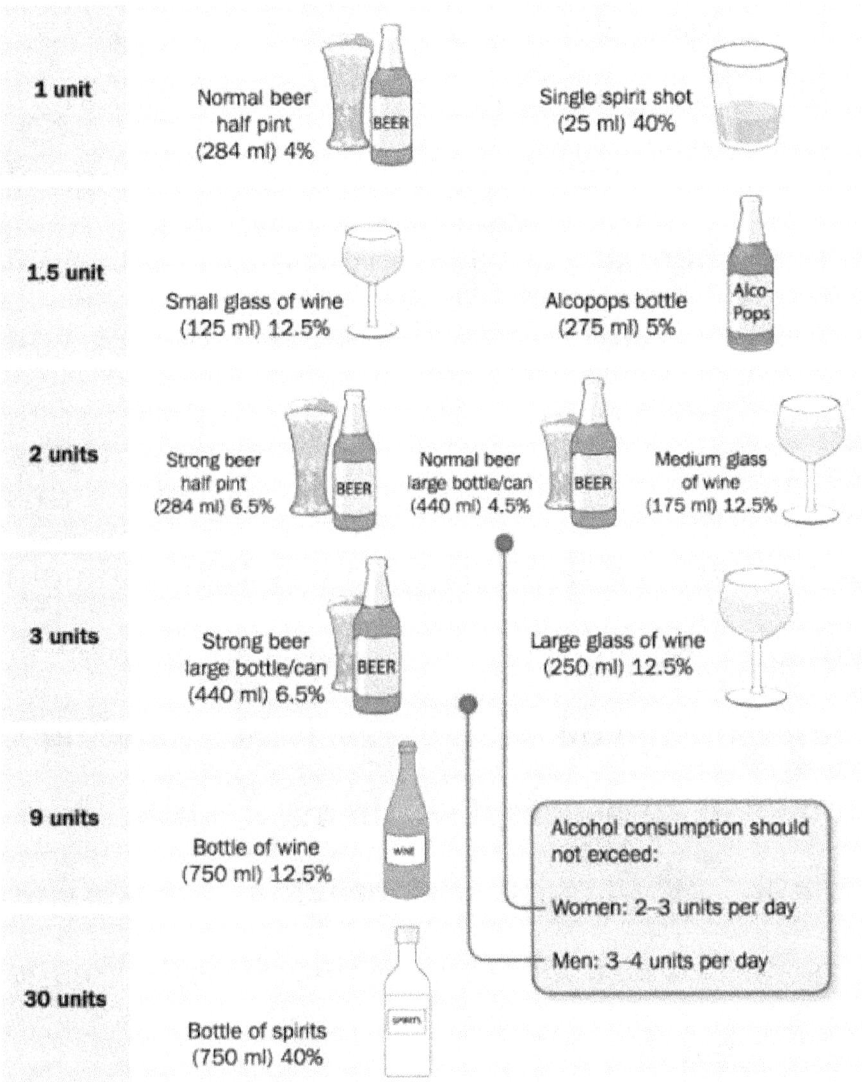

Day Twelve and Thirteen

The change plan

Even when you have committed to making a change, you still may have mixed feelings at times. There are days where a lot of confusion would becloud your mind and it makes you want to grow crazy. To avoid situations such as this Making a written "change plan" this will serve as a reminder strategy that will help you to strengthen your goals, recording reasons why you want to reach them, and how you plan to accomplish them. we have been able to set a goal in the previous week. This week and in the next two days, we will engage in the change plan.

A sample form is provided below. After filling it in, you can print it or email it to yourself to serve as a constant reminder.

THE CHANGE PLAN FORM

Goal: You can also just write down what you set as your goal in the previous week or (select one). This is very critical to continuing and finishing strong in your plans.

- I want to drink no more than ___ drink(s) on any day and no
- more than ___drink(s) per week (see low-risk drinking limits).
- I want to stop drinking.

Timing: I will start on this date: ___

Reasons: My most important reasons to make these changes are:____

Strategies: I will use these strategies:____

People: The people who can help me are (names and how they can help):___

Signs of success: I will know my plan is working if: (indicate notable signs)___

Possible roadblocks: Some things that might interfere—and how I'll handle them. (Make a list of all that applies)

Roadblocks:

We have talked about this as avoiding temptations so this more of an action plan. So fill out this plan and keep it where accessible.

Day Fourteen

Remake a list of Pros and cons

It's up to you as to whether and when to change your drinking. Other people may be able to help, but in the end, it's your decision. Weighing your pros and cons can help.

Pros: What are some reasons you might want to change your drinking?

Please check at least one pro.

- o To improve my health
- o To improve my relationships
- o To avoid hangovers
- o To do better at work or in school
- o To save money
- o To lose weight or get fit
- o To avoid more serious problems
- o To meet my standards

Cons: What are some possible barriers, or reasons you might not want to change your drinking?

Please check at least one con.

- I'd need another way to unwind.
- It helps me feel more at ease socially.
- I wouldn't fit in with some of my friends.
- Change can be hard.

Rate Your Pros

Now you rate your purposes for changing and attach their importance to you.

Purpose for changing	Rating
To improve my relationships	• Somewhat important • Fairly important • Important • Very important • Extremely important
To do better at work or in school	• Somewhat important • Fairly important • Important • Very important • Extremely important

To meet my standards	• Somewhat important • Fairly important • Important • Very important • Extremely important
To avoid more serious problems	• Somewhat important • Fairly important • Important • Very important • Extremely important

Exercise:

Do well to include other purposes you can think of and assign ratings to them.

Compare your pros and cons.

Is there a difference between where you are and where you want to be?

Although it can be challenging, it is possible to manage the difficulties, find healthy alternatives, and overcome the barriers to making a change.

WEEK THREE

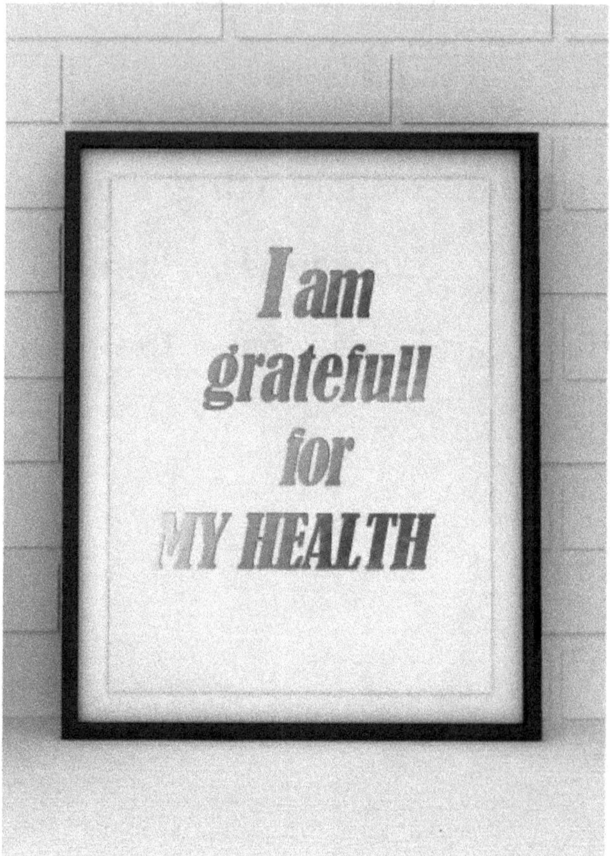

Whether you choose to tackle your alcohol addiction by going to rehab, getting therapy, or taking a self-directed treatment approach, support is essential. Don't try to go it alone. Recovering from alcohol addiction or abuse is much easier when you have people you can lean on for encouragement, comfort, and guidance.

Support can come from family members, friends, counsellors, other recovering alcoholics, your healthcare providers, and people from your faith community. Lean on close friends and family - Having the support of friends and family members is an invaluable asset in recovery.

If you're reluctant to turn to your loved ones because you've let them down before, consider going to couples counselling or family therapy.

Build a sober social network - If your previous social life revolved around alcohol, you may need to make some new connections. It's important to have sober friends who will support your recovery.

Try taking a class, joining a church or a civic group, volunteering, or attending events in your community. Make meetings a priority - Join a recovery support group, such as Alcoholics Anonymous (AA), and attend meetings regularly.

Spending time with people who understand exactly what you're going through can be very healing. You can also benefit from the shared experiences of the group members and learn what others have done to stay sober.

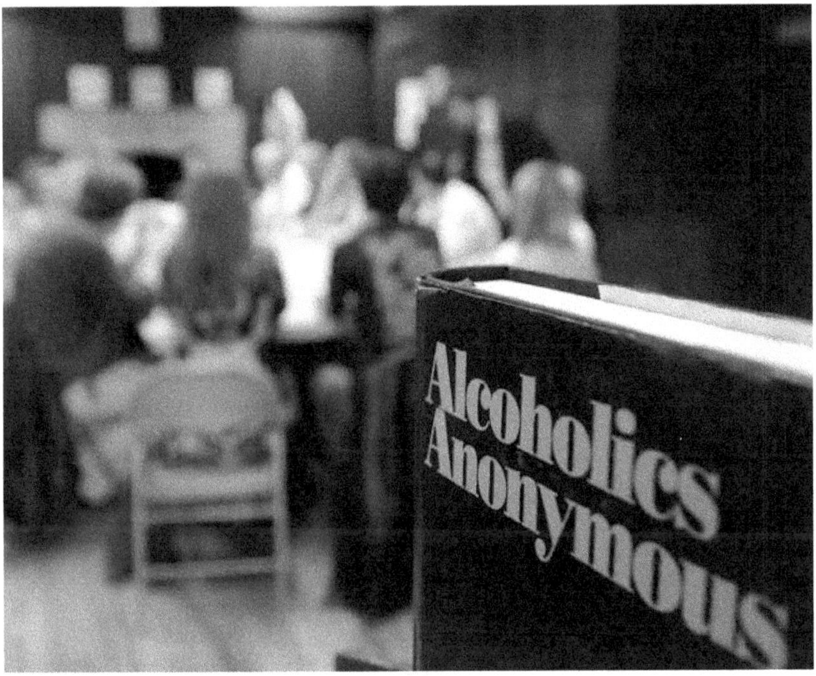
Alcoholics
Anonymous

DAY FIFTEEN TO TWENTY-ONE

You Need A Social Support

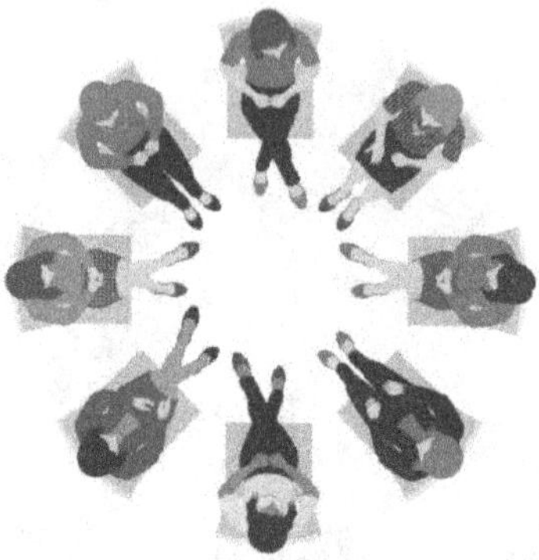

For most people asking for help can be difficult and it may translate to them not having their situation under control. The truth remains that whether you choose to tackle your alcohol addiction by going to rehab, getting therapy, or taking a self-directed treatment approach, support is essential and cannot be overemphasized.

Don't try to go through it alone, recovering from alcohol addiction or abuse is much easier when you have people you can lean on for encouragement, comfort, and guidance.

Support can come from family members, friends, counsellors, other recovering alcoholics, your healthcare providers, and people from your faith community.

Lean on close friends and family - Having the support of friends and family members is an invaluable asset in recovery. If you're reluctant to turn to your loved ones because you've let them down before, consider going to couples counselling or family therapy.

Build a sober social network - If your previous social life revolved around alcohol, you may need to make some new connections. It's important to have sober friends who will support your recovery.

Try taking a class, joining a church or a civic group, volunteering, or attending events in your community. Make meetings a priority - Join a recovery support group, such as Alcoholics Anonymous (AA), and attend meetings regularly. Spending time with people who understand exactly what you're going through can be very healing. You can also benefit from the shared experiences of the group members and learn what others have done to stay sober.

Here are some tips you can use to ask for help from anyone:

1. Write a letter or an email

You will be shocked at how many people would want to support you. As part of this week's exercise write a letter or send an email one each day to potential supporters, it may be to an online mentor, a religious leader, a role mother, or even your parents. The idea is to let your request out.

2. Ask for help from a medical professional

A drinking problem is a medical condition. Maybe it is called alcoholism or alcohol abuse, but sometimes a medical intervention might be a helpful solution and just the right step in the right direction. Book an appointment today with a professional to start your life-changing experience.

3. Talk to someone you trust

There is a level of satisfaction you get from knowing that someone is on your side and is willing to stand by your side through the hard times. Just having someone you can talk to will go a long way in helping you in achieving your drinking goals. Vulnerability comes from trust. There is a level of trust you have for a person or group of persons you are vulnerable bought to share some of your worst secrets with the having the confidence that there are no judgments, of your weaknesses won't be used against you in the future.

4. Look for people with similar issues or who has had a previous experience:

One who has been through a similar struggle as yours and has come out on the other side strong will always have a bit of better and first-hand advice. They likely remember what it was like to be where you are and will do what they can to ease your fears. You can ask them what worked for them and try to determine whether the same course of action would work well for you.

WEEK FOUR

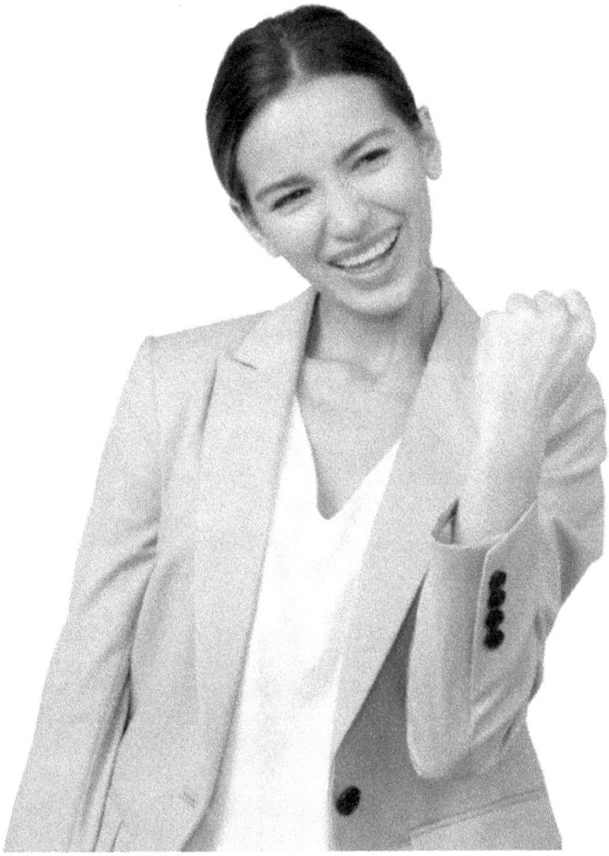

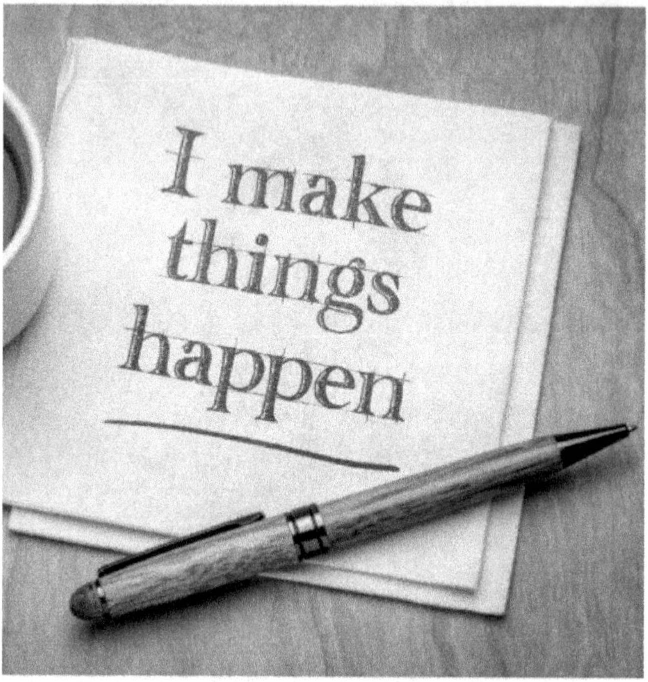
I make
things
happen

Marie has a made couple of good friends at her regular AA meetings- she needed to attend and her attendance was sent to her company- this and one of the many other requirements were to be fulfilled to keep her job and the contract. They were all the terms and conditions she accepted when the contract was awarded to her.

One of the days she was running late for her meetings. It was a weekday and she had closed late from work. She approached the bus station, and it took her over thirty minutes to get a taxi. Halfway into the journey, the driver realized he had a flat tyre and had to stop to fix it. By now Marie was already fuming with rage and cursing under her breath.

She felt like crying because her job depended on her attendance at these meeting, trying to figure out a solution she searched through her bag, and just as she was about to call Sophie to come to pick her up a neat Mercedes pulled up just after where her taxi was parked and asked if she wanted a lift. Marie did not know the stranger and did not even think twice about the offer, she just hopped in the car.

Charles was all shades of charming, from his neat and well-groomed haircut to his dress sense down to his taste in music—one need not to the told that he came from affluence. He asked her where she was heading to and she gave him the address. Coincidentally, the conference hall used for the meeting was not far from his destination.

Throughout the journey, they talked a lot about work and music. She tried as much as she can to avoid discussions concerning where she was going and her challenge. She considered it to be a turn-off. In less than 15 minutes, they arrived at her destination and she was very grateful and happy for this miracle. They exchanged numbers and he offered to come to pick her up after she was done. Marie was so charmed by this young man that deep down she wanted to see him again so she obliged his request.

– One hour later, they were in a lounge where he just finished meeting his client -

The waiter approached them to take their offer and she opted for water only, there were lots of spirits on the menu and she started feeling sad that she couldn't have one. It got worse when her date requested an alcoholic drink. She immediately excused herself and went to the ladies, where she tried to calm her nerves and practice her breathing exercise.

Charles was still at the table waiting for her as she stayed for so long. When she finally got back to the table, she apologizes for taking so much time- by then, their order had arrived and she was surprised to notice that Charles had changed his order to a non-alcoholic beverage. She was taking a back for a moment and had to ask why he changed his order.

He didn't want her to feel embarrassed as it was just the first time getting to know each other, but she insisted and he gave in. He explained that he noticed her reaction when he placed his order and when she excused herself to use the ladies her AA card fell. At this point, he handed her over the card. Marie looked flushed and embarrassed but he tried to calm her down and explain that he understands and will do all he can to support her.

In the next couple of days, we will try to build our Refusal skills and learn exercises that will help keep our urge at bay.

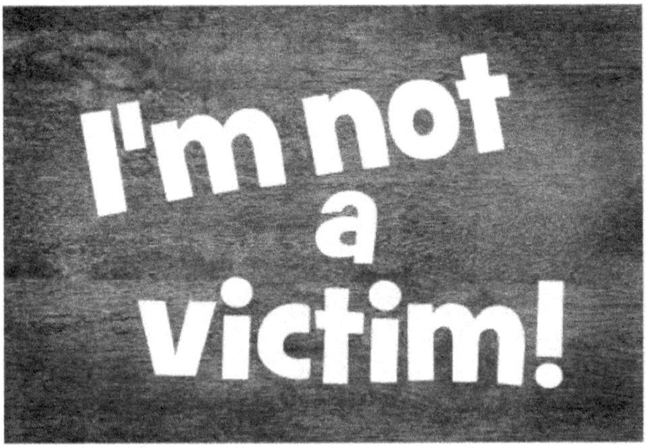

Not anymore!

DAY TWENTY-TWO TO TWENTY-FOUR

Building your drinking refusal Skill

Drinking Refusal Self-Efficacy Questionnaire

Direction:

The following questions ask you to describe your ability to handle drinking situations. Your answers will be your skill assessment so do well to answer as honestly as you can. The following pages contain a list of situations in which people may find themselves drinking alcohol. Please circle the number beside each statement that best describes how much you could resist drinking in each case.

I am very sure I could NOT resist drinking	I am most likely would NOT resist drinking	I probably could NOT resist drinking	I probably could resist drinking	I most likely could resist drinking	I am very sure I could resist drinking
1	2	3	4	5	6

1.	When I am watching TV	1	2	3	4	5	6
2	**When I am angry**	**1**	**2**	**3**	**4**	**5**	**6**
3	**When I am having lunch**	**1**	**2**	**3**	**4**	**5**	**6**
4	**When I am at a party**	**1**	**2**	**3**	**4**	**5**	**6**
5	**When I am on my way home from work**	**1**	**2**	**3**	**4**	**5**	**6**
6	**When someone offers me a drink**	**1**	**2**	**3**	**4**	**5**	**6**

7	**When I feel frustrated**	**1**	**2**	**3**	**4**	**5**	**6**
8	**When my partner is drinking**	**1**	**2**	**3**	**4**	**5**	**6**
9	**When I am worried**	**1**	**2**	**3**	**4**	**5**	**6**
10	**When I am by myself**	**1**	**2**	**3**	**4**	**5**	**6**
11	**When my friends are drinking**	**1**	**2**	**3**	**4**	**5**	**6**
12	**When I feel upset**	**1**	**2**	**3**	**4**	**5**	**6**
13	**When I have just finished playing sport**	**1**	**2**	**3**	**4**	**5**	**6**
14	**When I am at a nightclub or concert**	**1**	**2**	**3**	**4**	**5**	**6**
15	**When I am feeling down**	**1**	**2**	**3**	**4**	**5**	**6**
16	**When I first arrive home**	**1**	**2**	**3**	**4**	**5**	**6**
17	**When I feel nervous**	**1**	**2**	**3**	**4**	**5**	**6**

18	**When I feel sad**	**1**	**2**	**3**	**4**	**5**	**6**
19	**When I am listening to music or reading**	**1**	**2**	**3**	**4**	**5**	**6**

The above is a drinking refusal questionnaire and it will help you determine how you react to alcohol and situations that predispose you to drink. It will help you evaluate where you are at the moment with refusal.

Humans and then women are by nature social beings and being offered drinks in a social gathering will certainly occur, but developing a refusal skill will help you to stay at bay and not give in to temptations.

Below are some ways to help build your refusal skills

1. Know when to say "No":

Always be clear and assertive without hesitation. Many times a convincing "no" may suffice other times a tougher approach is required, In this case, don't flinch, maintain eye contact and be firm when declining an invitation to drink.

2. Suggesting alternatives to drinking: When hanging out with friends chose a location with fewer tendencies of assessing alcohol. For example, you can choose restaurants that are close to the playground or a school because these locations are less likely to stuck alcohol. Also, when placing your order it is always better to opt for a non-alcoholic beverage.

Practice:

1. Above is a drinking refusal skill efficacy questionnaire, fill it honestly by following the directions on the top of the form. This will give you a guide on how to set your strategies and where you are at the moment.

2. Now that you've seen some refusal techniques, take out time to come up with one or two techniques peculiar to you. For each day, come up with two (2) new approaches you would employ in refusing a drink and try to use them as often as possible.

DAY TWENTY-FIVE AND TWENTY-SIX

Practice 'Urge surfing'

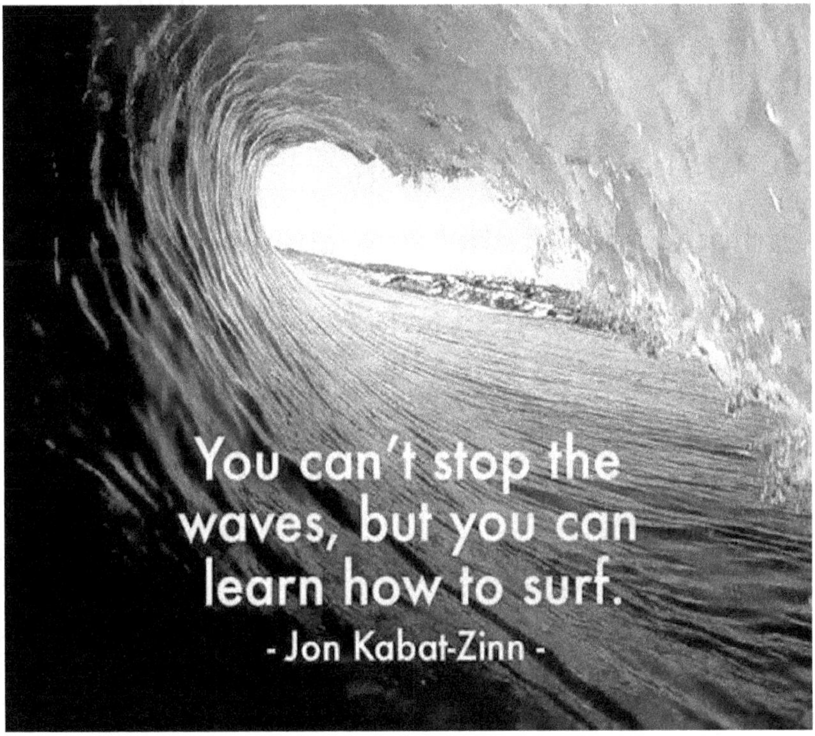

Urge surfing has been proven to help break unhelpful habits and we will employ this with drinking habits.

what is urge surfing and how it works?

The term "Urge surfing" was coined by clinical psychologist Alan Marlatt in his book In his book, *Relapse Prevention: Maintenance Strategies in the Treatment of Addictive Behaviors* (first published in 1985 and revised in 2005). He described urge surfing as an imaging technique used in helping clients gain control over impulses to use drugs or alcohol.

The technique involves first teaching the client to label internal sensations and cognitive preoccupations as an urge, after which they strive to foster an attitude of detachment from that urge.

Cravings are always temporary and that is why this technique proves helpful. Although the time it takes for an urge to last varies depending on the type of craving and the coping mechanism, most research suggests that the urge tends to subside after 30minutes. Another noteworthy fact is that each time you outlast a craving, the less frequent and intense it becomes in the future.

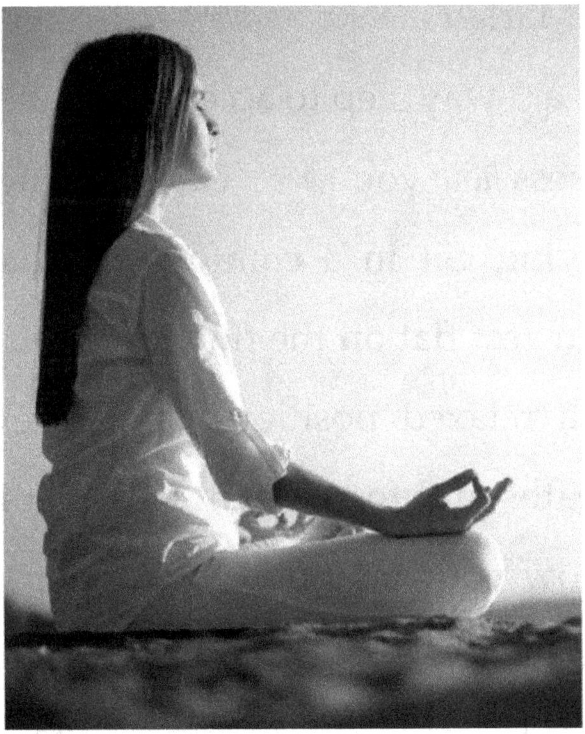

Steps to Surf urging

Carefully follow the steps below to get your urge under control, try this for these few days and watch yourself getting control.

Step 1: Accept that urges will occur

"The focus is on identifying and accepting the urge, not acting on the urge or attempting to fight it."

– Alan Marlatt

Below is a 3-way step to accept your urge

- Assess *how* you're experiencing the craving. Sit in a comfortable chair with your feet flat on the floor and your hands in a relaxed position. Take a few deep breaths and focus your attention inward. Allow your attention to wander through your body. Notice the part of your body where you're experiencing the craving and what the sensations are like. Tell yourself what it feels like. For example, "My craving is in my mouth and nose and my stomach."

- Focus on one area where you're experiencing the urge: How do the sensations in that area feel? For example, perhaps you feel hot, cold, tingly, or numb? Are your muscles tense or relaxed? How large an area is involved? Describe the sensations to yourself and any changes that occur. "My mouth feels dry and parched. There is tension in my lips and tongue. I keep swallowing. As I exhale, I can imagine the smell and tingle of a drink."

Repeat on each part of your body that's experiencing the craving: What changes occur in the sensations? Notice how the urge comes and goes. You'll likely notice that after a few minutes the craving has gone. The purpose of urge surfing is not to make cravings disappear, but to experience them in a new way. However, with practice, you'll learn how to ride your cravings out until they go away naturally.

Step 2: Notice when an urge arises (Record your urge symptoms)

Identifying what triggers your urge will help you to be better prepared for handling it instead of engaging in your drinking habits without thinking.

Practice

Try to identify these "cues" in your drink habit, you can even think of others:

Do you engage in your habit at a particular time of the day or in a certain place?

Is there an emotion that triggers your habit?

Does a person in your life prompt your habit?

Once you know how to recognize your urge then you are halfway there. follow-through to step 3.

Step 3: Resist from acting on your urge.

If you followed the previous step you should have been able to recognize an urge. Once you've noticed that symptom, try not to act upon it.

knowing how difficult this step could be you might want to start by delaying the habit, rather than resisting it entirely.

Practice

Once urge has been identified in any of the symptoms peculiar to you, delay the habit for a couple of minutes say five minutes. Next time, extend the time to seven minutes. Then ten and gradually but consistently it ceases to become an urge.

Step 4: Visualize your urge as a "wave"

Visualizing your urge as a wave can help in controlling how you deal with it. Picture yourself on a surfboard with the wave being your drive instead. Instead of fighting it flow with it and watch how it gradually reduces its intensity as it approaches the shore. Visualize this and feel your urge's intensity diminish.

Step 5: Focus on your breath

When you feel your urge intensify, switch your focus to your breathing. Take a few deep breaths, inhale and exhale. During each exhales, purse your lips like you want to blow a whistle so it lasts longer. Do this for 20seconds.

DAY TWENTY-SEVEN AND TWENTY-EIGHT

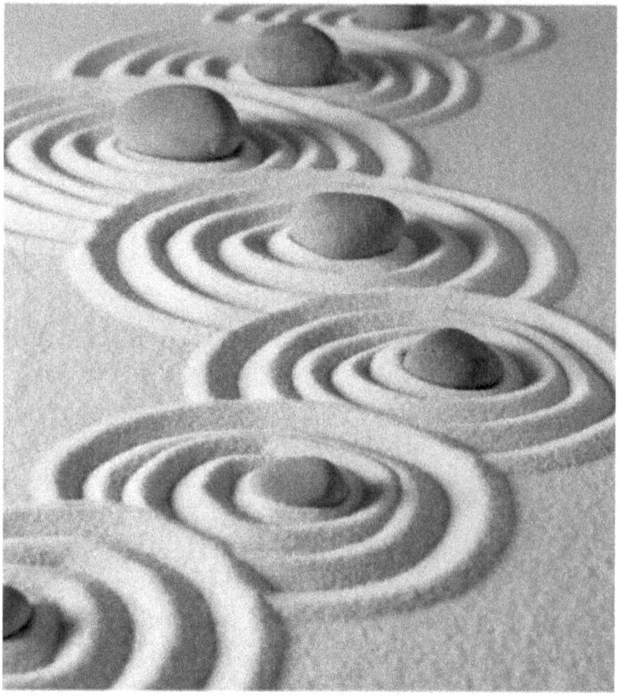

Find new meaning in life while getting sober is an important first step, it is only the beginning of your recovery from alcohol addiction or heavy drinking. Rehab or professional treatment can get you started on the road to recovery, but to stay alcohol-free for the long term, you'll need to build a new, meaningful life where drinking no longer has a place.

Five steps to a sober lifestyle

1. Take care of yourself: To prevent mood swings and combat cravings, concentrate on eating right and getting plenty of sleep.
2. Exercise is also key: it releases endorphins, relieves stress, and promotes emotional well-being. Build your support network. Surround yourself with positive influences and people who make you feel good about yourself. The more you're invested in other people and your community, the more you have to lose—which will help you stay motivated and on the recovery track. Develop new activities and interests.
3. Find new hobbies, volunteer activities, or work that gives you a sense of meaning

and purpose. When you're doing things you find fulfilling, you'll feel better about yourself and drinking will hold less appeal.

4. Continue treatment: Your chances of staying sober improve if you are participating in a support group like Alcoholics Anonymous, have a sponsor or are involved in therapy or an outpatient treatment program.
5. Healthily deal with stress: Alcohol abuse is often a misguided attempt to manage stress. Find healthier ways to keep your stress level in checks, such as exercising, meditating, or practising breathing exercises or other relaxation techniques.

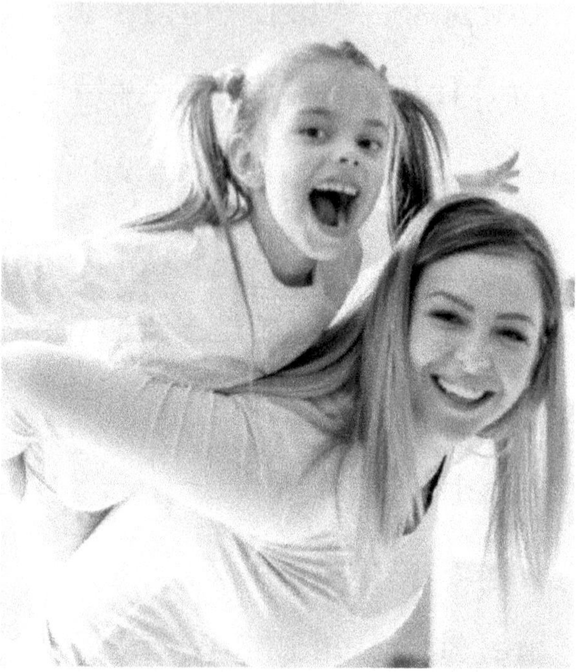

Introduction:

The majority of people already know that smoking is harmful to their health. On the other hand, are you aware of how harmful smoking is? Tobacco includes nicotine, a highly addictive substance that makes quitting smoking difficult. Besides nicotine, tobacco products also include a number of toxic and hazardous chemicals that may lead to illness and death. Did you know that out of 1000 smokers (age 30), a quarter (250!) will die of smoking-related illnesses before reaching middle age, another quarter will die prematurely from smoking-related illnesses shortly after retirement age, and a third group will develop debilitating chronic illnesses as a result of their smoking? Most people are unaware that the chances of being ill as a consequence of smoking are really very high, yet when the statistics are crunched, that is exactly what you get. For many individuals, realising the serious health risks connected with smoking is the driving force behind their decision to stop.

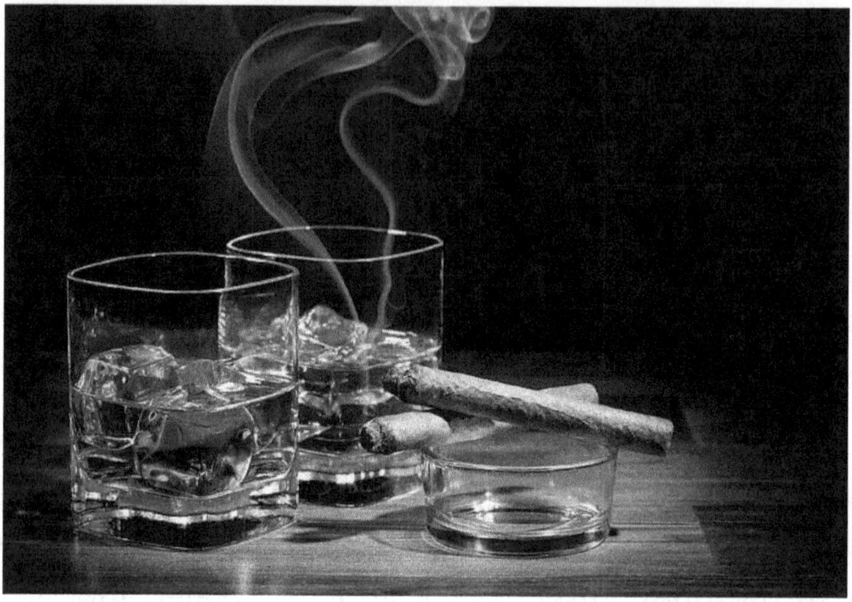

During the 1990s, smoking prevalence rose by almost 30% among college students, according to the American Cancer Society (ACS).

Even though the vast majority of college students begin smoking before the age of 18, new research indicates that a significant proportion of undergraduates report starting to smoke while in college.

Among undergraduate students enrolled at a major public institution in the southwestern United States, this research looked at the use of alcohol and tobacco together and the connection between alcohol consumption and the start of smoking among a sample of undergraduate students.

For this research, we divided participants into three groups based on their smoking status: never smokers (n=777), experimenters (n=158), and smokers (n=178).

There was a statistically significant difference between experimenters and smokers on both of these measures of consumption when compared to never smokers. However, there was no statistically significant difference between experimenters and smokers when it came to one of these consumption measures in the past two weeks.

After adjusting for demographic and other drug use variables, the findings of two multinomial logistic regression models revealed that alcohol intake and drinking frequency measures were substantially related to being an experimenter or a smoker.

In the results of logistic regression analysis, it was discovered that there was a statistically significant connection between the previous year's drinking frequency and smoking start among respondents who stated that they had not smoked at all in the 12 months before their survey participation.

The impact of alcohol intake on the start of smoking among college students is addressed in this article.

History of Drinking

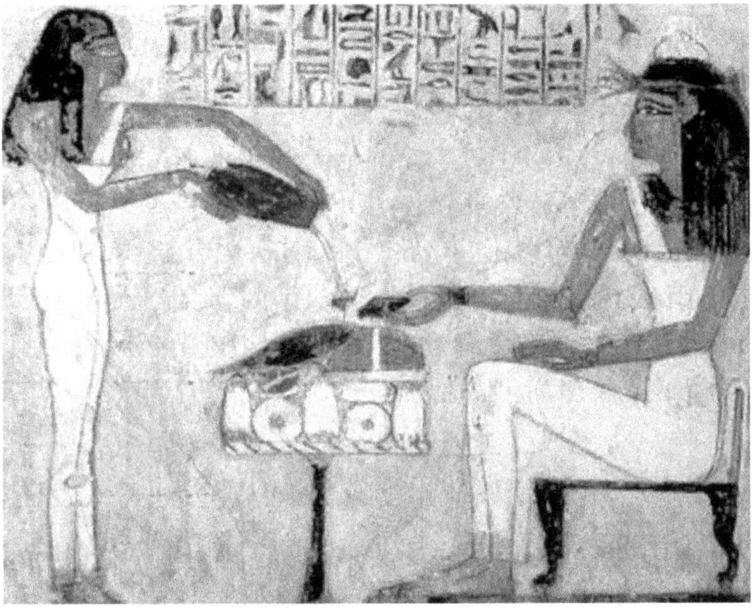

The following overview of drinking's history examines the varied functions that alcohol has played in various societies.

Ancient Time

People have seen alcohol as a nourishing and comforting drug throughout history. Alcohol has even been regarded to have supernatural properties in many nations and cultures. One of the first things Noah did after the flood, according to the Bible, was to cultivate a vineyard (Genesis 9:21). The importance of alcohol is reflected in many mythology and religious beliefs. The ancient Egyptians thought that Osiris, the great deity, taught them how to manufacture beer, a liquid that was both spiritually and nutritionally important to them. Beer was buried and presented to the gods in royal graves. Wine was consumed as a form of worship by the Greeks. The Greeks thought that the deity Dionysus had given them wine. Bacchus was supposed to be both the creator and the constant presence of wine in Roman times. Mayahuel, the Aztec goddess, was said to have taught them how to produce a mild beer from the sap of the century plant. Beer is an essential part of many Indians' diets to this day.

Early wines and beers were not at all like the beverages we enjoy today. Until about 1700, the majority of wines and beers were black, sediment-laden, and of variable quality. Homebrew beers were usually very nutritious, but they only lasted a few days before going sour. Homemade wines were low in vitamins and minerals, but they could be stored for a long time if properly preserved.

Although it is impossible to establish when or where Homo sapiens first tried alcohol, chemical analysis of residues found in pots dating from 3500 B.C.E. suggests that wine was already being prepared in Mesopotamia from grapes (now Iraq). Alcohol is almost as old as farming as a result of this discovery. In truth, beer and bread were initially made from the same components in the same region at around the same time. We don't know much about how people gradually learned to control fermentation, blend drinks, and store and ship them in methods that preserved them from spoiling. We have learned about how commodities were carried from one place to another during ancient times by studying the varied designs of wine cups from various regions.

The Hebrews' religious customs in around 500 B.C.E. were very different from those of other nations. The Hebrews drank wine in holy family rites, but they also stressed temperance, or drinking in little amounts and at specific times. This tendency continues into the twenty-first century, and devout Jews' drinking is frequently distinguished from that of their neighbours. Early Christians, many of whom were Jews, lauded wine for its health and social benefits while condemning intoxication. The Bible provides numerous allusions to drinking in a good light. The solemn celebration of the Eucharist, or Holy Communion, which is a key practise in many Christian denominations, extends Jesus' choice of wine to signify his blood into the twenty-first century.

Although little is known about ancient Africa, mild fermented home brews (such as banana beer) were popular, as they were in Latin America. We know the most about Asia from China, where grain-based beer and wine were used in ceremonies, dedicated to the gods, and included in royal tombs as early as 2000 B.C.E. Drinking had clearly positive connotations for early peoples, as it does for many non-Western communities today.

Between 1000 and 1500

During the middle Ages, Christianity and Islam spread swiftly. People began to form national groups about this time as well. The civilizations of these rising nations vary, and each culture had its own preferences for drinks and drinking styles. Homebrewed beer was a staple of the diet for peasants and handicrafts. Nobles chastised impoverished people for their excessive drinking, while they themselves ate and drank lavishly. Taverns became key social centres in towns and villages, and the elite often decried them as harmful to religion, political stability, and family life.

During this time, hops were added, which improved the flavour and durability of beer. Wine became even more popular in Italy and France, both as a food and as a commodity. Since around 800, Arabs have known how to distil spirits (such as whiskey, brandy, and other drinks that are now commonly referred to as hard liquor). Until before 1200, that technology was controlled by a tiny group of religious leaders, physicians, and alchemists in Europe. They sold the spirits they made as beverages as a luxury item and for medicinal purposes.

Drinking and inebriation were celebrated as techniques to alter consciousness among populations across northern Africa and much of Asia. Most Africans and Asians became temperate and sometimes abstinent as the doctrines of Islam, Buddha, and Confucius spread. Both China and India had periods of prohibition during which alcohol consumption was prohibited. Some castes, or social classes, in Hinduism consumed booze as a sacred ceremony. Drinking was frowned upon by others.

European sea exploration expanded during the Renaissance. Europeans met civilizations and tribal peoples who had long colonised North, Central, and South America. Although a wide range of beers and other fermented brews were essential in Mexico as delicacies, sacrifices to the gods, and direct ways to reach religious ecstasy, alcoholic beverages appear to have been completely unknown north of Mexico.

From 1500 to 1800

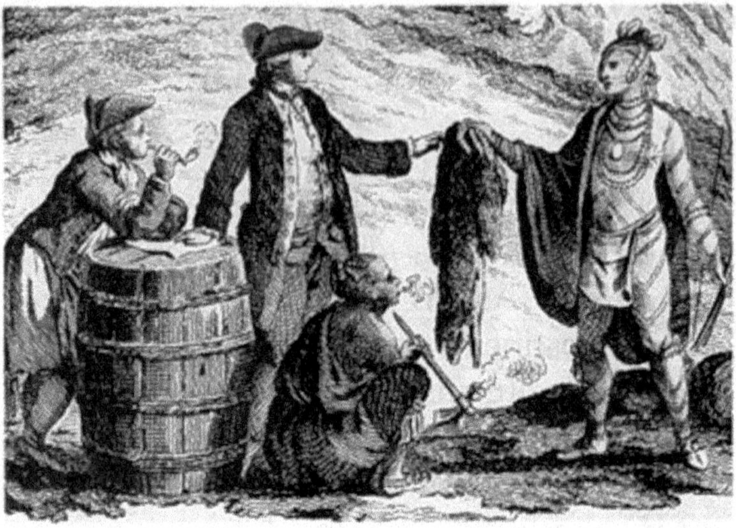

The Protestant Reformation had an impact on people's lives all around Europe. One such shift was the perception that intoxication was a bad way to celebrate. Long-term heavy drinking was frowned upon by the believers. Despite this, public drinking facilities became key town gathering places where workers could catch up on the latest news, gossip, and play games. The nobility began to drink brandies, and champagne, as well as numerous cordials and liqueurs, was introduced as a luxury beverage. As technology and quality control increased, brewing and winemaking became big enterprises.

The Spanish and Portuguese conquistadors (conquerors) discovered that indigenous peoples in Latin America and parts of North America already had home brews that were vital to them for food, medicine, and religious purposes. Beer provided a substantial amount of the Aztecs' nutritional diet, but only priests and old men were permitted to be intoxicated. As part of their rain ceremony, the Yaqui (in what is now Arizona) produced cactus wine. Spanish and Portuguese colonial authorities attempted to implement rules and regulations prohibiting the consumption and production of alcohol, but these prohibitions were inconsistently enforced. Liquor quickly became an essential item as merchants from several places fought for commerce with the various Native American groups of North America.

Rum, distilled from West Indian sugar output, became a major item in international trade in the colonies that subsequently formed the United States. Captive black Africans were carried to the West Indies to be sold as slaves in the Triangle Trade. Many laboured on plantations, producing not only refined sugar, a sweet and valuable new food, but also molasses, which was brought to New England in large quantities. Molasses was made into rum by distillers in the area, which was then carried to West Africa to be traded for more slaves.

However, after the American Revolution (1775-1783), the commerce triangle was disrupted, and North Americans began making whiskey. Farmers east of the Mississippi River, along the frontier at the time, were ready to make money by distilling their surplus corn into whiskey. In 1790, a federal tax on whiskey was introduced to assist pay off the nascent United States' debt. The new tax enraged the producing farmers so much that they banded together to fight it. The Whiskey Rebellion of 1794 caused the new federal government to call up the militia (federal troops) for the first time in order to quell the uprising. Around the same time, Benjamin Rush, a well-known physician and signer of the Declaration of Independence, began a crusade against long-term heavy drinking, claiming that it was harmful to one's health.

During the 1800s,

Beer, wine, and distilled liquor became popular throughout Europe throughout the Industrial Revolution. Products were sold to countries all around the world by businesses and industries. Drinking became a desirable leisure activity as a new middle class arose with more time and money to spend. For many, it was a welcome break from the suffocating atmosphere of the office.

Alcohol began to lose a lot of its religious significance about this time. It was regarded by certain Protestant groups and Catholic priests to be the cause of crime, family disintegration, unemployment, and other social issues. Long-term heavy drinking was also connected to sickness by certain doctors and scholars, though liquor remained a significant part of medicine for certain purposes. Herbs soaked in alcohol were used to make many medicines. In reality, most patent medicines promoted for every imaginable ailment contained alcohol. These medicines, which were meant to ease colicky newborns, also targeted babies. Little was known about how or why some people had problems with alcohol while others did not.

A wave of religious activity swept over the United States in the early 1800s, including concerns about the use of alcohol. By 1850, a dozen states had outlawed the manufacture of alcoholic beverages. When religious tensions subsided, these municipal prohibition ordinances were finally overturned. The public became captivated with hard-drinking cowboys, miners, lumberjacks, and other colourful characters of the expanding frontier after the Civil War (1861–1865). As the United States grew westward, wealth became an essential indicator of social standing. By serving exclusively those from a certain economic class, certain public drinking places represented social prestige or importance.

Toward the end of the 1800s, a new anti-alcohol movement emerged. Protestants in northern states like New York and Massachusetts perceived a significant influx of immigrants, many of whom were Catholics, as a threat. These new Catholic immigrants competed for jobs and posed a threat to Protestant control of politics, governance, and mainstream ideals, which had been in place for decades. Protestants scorned the newcomers' drinking habits, urging them to practise "clean living." Meanwhile, Native American populations were being driven off their lands and, in some cases, wiped altogether. In books and news articles, the stereotype of the intoxicated Indian began to emerge. Many Indians stayed abstinent in fact.

The Twentieth Century

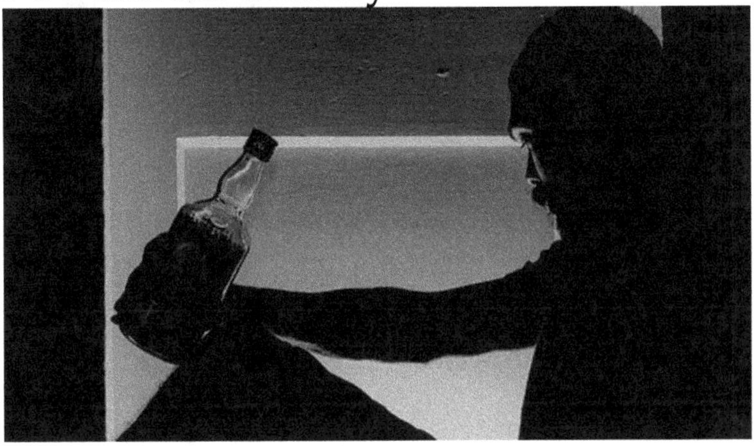

Many notable changes occurred in daily living during the twentieth century. Pasteurization, mass production, commercial canning and bottling, and speedy transportation are only a few of the advances that have enhanced the conditions for producing and selling alcohol. At the same time, new views about the government's role in public health and social welfare evolved. As a result of these views, we now expect the government to impose restrictions on drinking and the sale of alcohol.

The statewide prohibition of alcohol in the United States was enacted in 1919 as a result of a mixture of religious objections to drinking and unfounded medical assertions about its risks. The Constitution's Eighteenth Amendment prohibited commercial sales of alcohol but made no mention of drinking or possession. At initially, there was very little alcohol manufacture at home and very little smuggling. However, unauthorized sources finally surfaced.

Moonshiners were individuals who illegally distilled booze, while bootleggers were those who trafficked it within the United States or from overseas. Cities and towns sprouted speakeasies, or secret bars and cocktail lounges, and drinking became even more fashionable than before prohibition. Dealing in alcohol made some business owners extremely wealthy. Meanwhile, the government was losing money due to the loss of alcohol taxes.

The stock market fall of 1929 was followed by huge unemployment, an agricultural crisis, and global economic despair. Prohibition enraged Americans, and some of the same powerful people who had pushed for it now agitated for its repeal. In 1933, the Twenty-first Amendment, the first and only repeal of the United States Constitution, repealed federal prohibition. The states were given the authority to set their own retail sales regulations. Many states were declared dry, which meant that no booze could be sold within their borders. Others gave counties or towns the authority to determine whether or not to allow alcohol.

From the end of prohibition until the early 1980s, American consumption of all alcoholic beverages climbed gradually, with a sharp spike following World War II (1939–1945). Alcoholics Anonymous was founded in the mid-twentieth century by a group of people who were addicted to alcohol (AA). AA has developed into an international fellowship of people whose primary goal is to avoid drinking. Scientists began examining the effects of alcohol in the mid-twentieth century, and our understanding has evolved significantly since then. Alcoholism is now seen as a sickness rather than a moral issue by the general people.

Spirits sales began to decline around 1980 and have since continued to decline. Wine sales peaked a few years later and have since gradually declined; beer sales appear to have peaked even more recently. Despite greater advertising, these decreases happened. The decline in alcohol use could be attributed to a widespread belief in a healthy lifestyle that emphasises physical activity and a balanced diet.

Risk Factors for Alcoholism

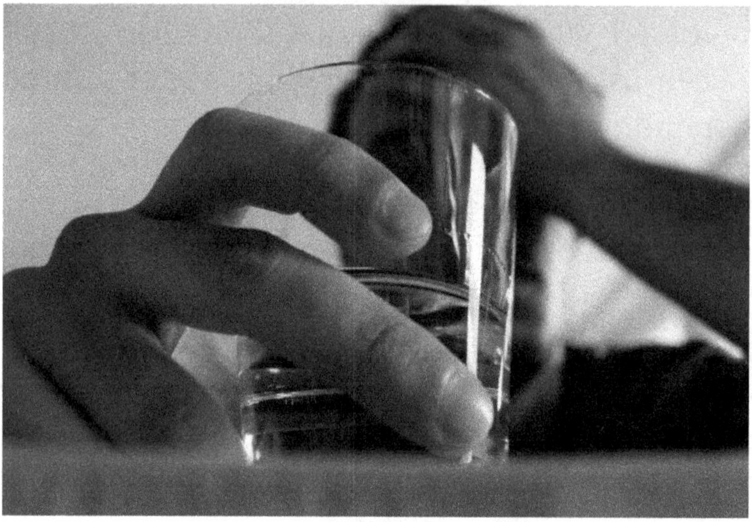

There are numerous risk factors associated with the development of alcoholism. Alcoholism risk factors do not guarantee that you will develop a drinking problem; rather, they should serve as a preventative step. If you have at least one risk factor, speak with a medical practitioner about alcoholism warning signs and resources for prevention. The following are some basic risk factors for alcohol abuse:

- **Beginning to Drink at a Young Age**

Drinking too much alcohol at a young age can lead to problems later in life, especially in your 20s and 30s. This is especially true when teens binge drinking on a regular basis. While early drinking can raise the likelihood of alcohol abuse, alcoholism can affect anyone at any age.

- **Alcohol Addiction in the Family**

Growing up with relatives and close family members who suffer from the negative consequences of consuming alcohol raises the likelihood of alcohol abuse in future generations. When you're around by people who drink excessively, you'll notice how people use alcohol differently and fall to bad habits.

- **Peer Influence**

When a partner or close companion drinks once in a while, you may be more inclined to join them. Surrendering to peer pressure can lead to drinking problems, as well as a slew of other unintended consequences of excessive alcohol consumption. Rather than drinking, volunteer to be a designated driver.

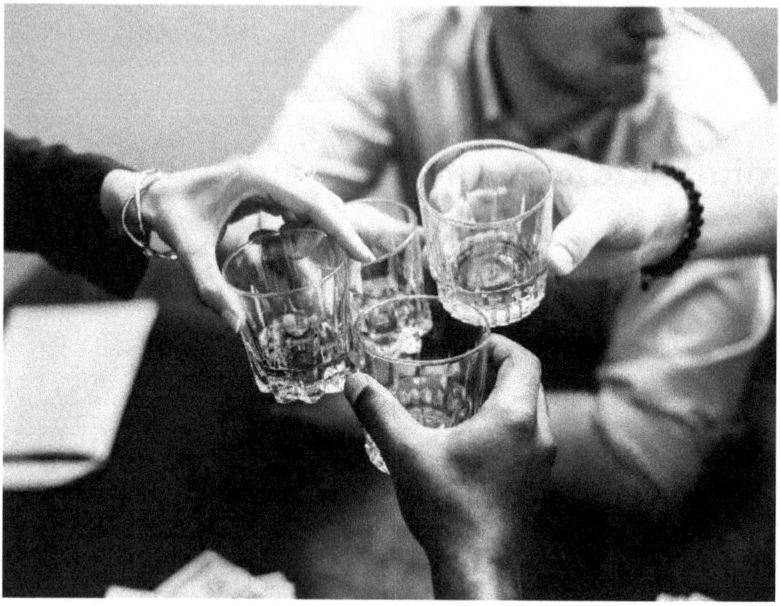

• Drinking a lot of alcohol over a long period of time

When excessive drinking becomes a pattern, you greatly increase your chances of developing an alcohol-related problem. The more you drink, the more your body develops an alcohol resistance. Resilience means that you'll need more alcohol to get the same affects you used to get with less.

• Combining Alcohol with Other Substances

Drinking alcohol to amplify or come down from the high of other substances, such as prescription opioids, benzodiazepines, or cocaine, is a form of polysubstance addiction that raises the risk of developing a true alcohol problem.

When alcohol is combined with other drugs - including those prescribed by a doctor - it can result in genuine well-being if proper precautions are not taken. Mixing alcohol with opioids, or even antidepressants or anxiety medications, for example, can result in undesirable side effects such as increased drowsiness, respiratory depression, and memory blackouts at high dosages.

- **Binge Consumption**

Binge drinking, which entails consuming a large amount of alcohol in a short period of time, is also a risk factor for alcoholism. This entails drinking at least five drinks in a single setting for men, and at least four for women.

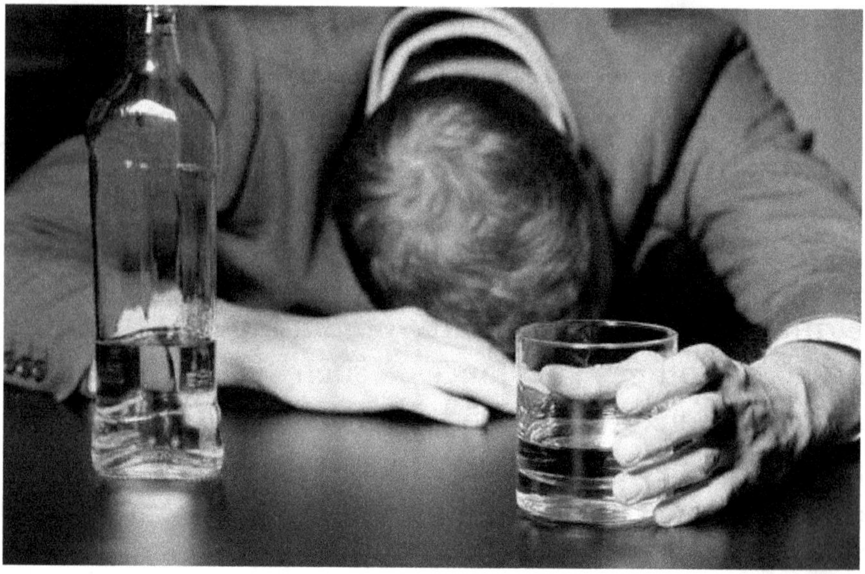

Young individuals between the ages of 18 and 34 drinking at this level on a regular basis. It's no coincidence that a large number of people this age are attending college and are likely to become engaged in "party culture."

The Effects of Parental Alcoholism on Children

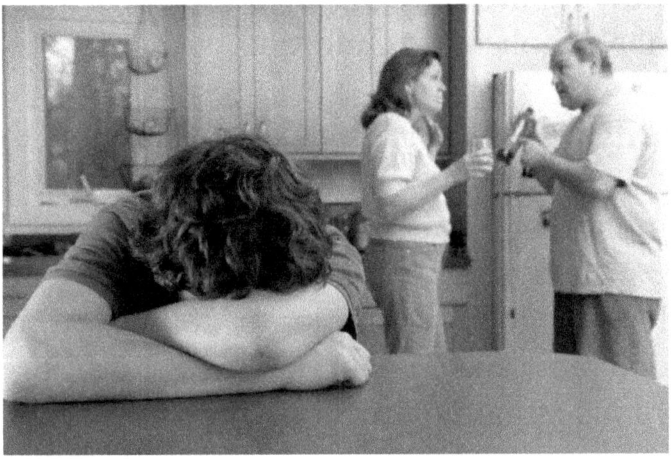

Many persons suffering from alcoholism have the misperception that their drinking has no impact on others. Of course, this isn't the case, and children with alcoholic parents are among the most vulnerable.

After reading about the effects of alcoholism on children now and in maturity, parents battling with alcoholism may be startled or alarmed. Their children, on the other hand, may take comfort in understanding what factors may have contributed to some of the problems they face now.

- **Psychiatric and Emotional Consequences**

Unfortunately, the consequences of growing up in an environment where alcoholism is prevalent can be so severe that they can last a lifetime, impacting how children and adults perceive themselves and others, participate in relationships, and more.

The following are only a few of the consequences of parental alcoholism on children.

- **Inability to Regain a Sense of Normalcy**

Adult offspring of alcoholics may have to assume what it means to be "normal" because they may not have had a good example to follow from their childhood and may never have had traditional or harmonious family interactions.

As a result, many people will feel conflicted, puzzled, and self-conscious when they learn that drinking is not common in other families.

- **Problems with Trust**

Adult offspring of alcoholics might suffer major trust issues after growing up in an environment where denial, lying, and concealing secrets may have been the norm. They've learned through broken promises in the past that trusting someone will backfire in the future.

Adult children may develop a phobia of all angry people if their alcoholic parent was harsh or abusive when they were intoxicated. They may spend their entire lives avoiding any type of disagreement or confrontation, fearing that it would turn violent.

- **Judge Them in a Cruel and Inhumane Way**

Some adult children of alcoholics take themselves quite seriously and find it extremely difficult to relax. They may have minimal self-worth and low self-esteem as a result of their upbringing, and they may develop severe feelings of inadequacy.

Children with an alcoholic father may believe they are different from other people and so unworthy of love. As a result, they may avoid social situations, find it difficult to make acquaintances, and isolate themselves.

- **Constantly seek other people's approval**

Some adult offspring of alcoholics continuously seek acceptance from others, in addition to criticizing themselves too harshly.

They can become people-pleasers who are shattered if someone is dissatisfied with them and live in constant fear of criticism.

Many children from alcoholic homes become overly responsible or perfectionists, and can become overachievers or workaholics, perhaps to avoid criticism or the wrath of their alcoholic father. On the other hand, it is fairly uncommon for someone to go in the opposite direction, imitating the same negative behaviors that they may have experienced as a youngster.

Factors that Contribute to Alcoholism

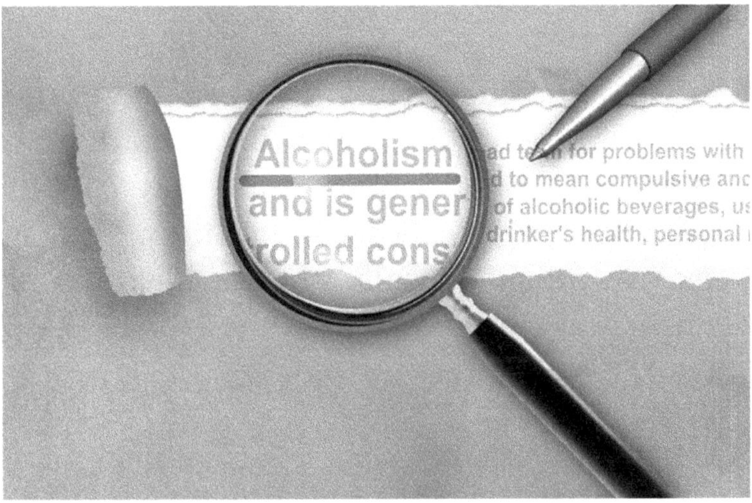

Alcohol abuse can be exacerbated by a variety of causes. People may turn to alcohol for a variety of reasons and eventually develop a drinking addiction. Drinking during painful times, such as a family tragedy or a job loss, might potentially lead to long-term alcohol abuse. While there are many reasons why people begin drinking, the following are some of the most common:

- **Stress relief**

Relying on alcohol to cope with everyday difficulties can increase the risk of developing alcoholism. Drinking promotes emotions of pleasure since alcohol is a depressive and sedative. Frequent drinking, on the other hand, increases tolerance, needing you to consume more alcohol to attain the same benefits.

- **Have a nice time**

Some people find that drinking alcohol gives them a respite from reality. It provides respite from underlying concerns that your mind may be striving to avoid. However, drinking to get through the day or week can quickly escalate into a major drinking problem.

- **Dealing with grief**

Losing a family member or a friend can be emotionally, physically, and mentally draining. Alcohol can help you cope with your sadness and is commonly used to help people get through difficult situations. Even momentarily relying on alcohol can lead to a drinking problem.

- **Become anxiety-free**

Some people are naturally anxious, which causes them to worry all of the time. Drinking decreases inhibitions and makes people feel more at ease in social circumstances. However, this can lead to addictive behaviors over time.

- **Inability to connect**

Many people drink because they don't feel connected to others enough. They assume that drinking alcohol will help them fill the emptiness or make it easier to form new ties. In most cases, however, the opposite is true.

- **Shame**

For many people, shame is one of the hardest feelings to deal with, as well as one of the most traumatic. While alcohol can momentarily disguise shame with false feelings, it also leads to many people engaging in risky or dumb activities that can lead to even more shame, which can lead to a downward spiral.

- **Trauma**

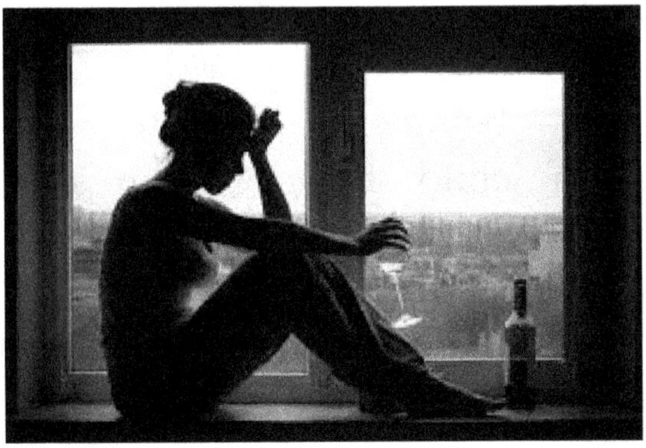

Almost every patient in a treatment center for alcoholism has experienced some kind of trauma. There are various types of trauma, but they are all terrible occurrences in which the sufferer was not accompanied by an empathic witness. Unresolved trauma is a major factor in many people's rehabilitation.

Why Are Children of Alcoholics Fearful of Angry People?

When they drink, alcoholics can become cruel and abusive. As a result, their children may grow up to be afraid of angry people. Even the appearance of conflict or disagreement can cause anxiety since there is a fear that the situation could escalate into wrath or violence.

Although fear of angry people is a common trait among adult children of alcoholics, it can also occur in children who grew up with a toxic (but not alcoholic) parent (such as those with cluster B personality disorders like narcissistic personality disorder) and were subjected to physical, psychological, or sexual abuse.

What effect does being exposed to angry and abusive conduct as a child have on an adult child's relationships when they are later exposed to anger? Understanding the meaning of your feelings may help you prevent maladaptive habits that may influence you long after the abuse you experienced as a child.

HOW Children of Alcoholics Might React When They're Angry

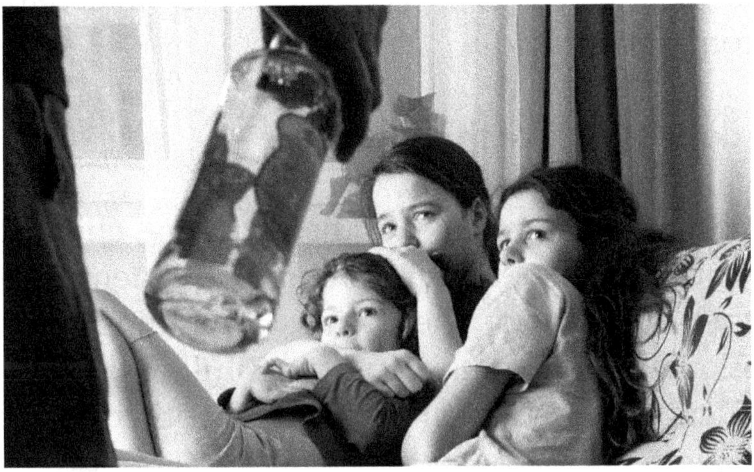

While being around angry and poisonous people can cause anxiety in adult offspring of alcoholics, the methods in which this presents itself can differ. Some of these habits, such as a strong hatred of yelling and screaming, may appear to be self-evident. Others, like being a people pleaser and a fixer, are less evident, but no less difficult.

Many adult children of alcoholics and toxic parents may not be aware that they are afraid of angry people, but they may recognise some of the defence mechanisms adopted by children to cope with such dread.

When these behaviours are ignored, one major issue is that they might lead to people pursuing hazardous relationships in the future. Some of the characteristics common among adult offspring of alcoholics, for example, can make them a target for bullies and a magnet for abusive people. Let's look at some of these behaviours that can lead to maladaptive outcomes in later life.

- **A desire to make things better**

Even though an issue is not theirs to cure, children of alcoholics and toxic parents frequently feel compelled to do so. The desire to "fix things" can be emotionally demanding and stressful, and it's often pointless because we can't actually fix other people.

This is how one woman characterized her need to correct things:

"I'll have to take care of it. If someone is angry with me, I get worried and feel compelled to rectify it right away. I put myself in victim roles or convince myself that I don't deserve aid because my circumstances aren't as awful as others'. I'm constantly feeling lonely and depressed."

Women are affected differently by an alcoholic father than men, and they may be more likely to become "fixers." In the case of the oldest daughter, this is especially true. Many adult children describe trouble having fun in their life as a result of their drive to "fix things."

It can take many years for adult children to be able to take a step back and realise that they are not responsible for another person's problems. However, doing so may be extremely liberating, and adult children who have fought to overcome their urge to fix things frequently express how much "lighter" they feel.

Unfortunately, toxic people are frequently only too willing to delegate their problems to others. To put it another way, if change is to occur, it must begin with you.

- **Intolerance of screams and yelling**

Adult children can be traumatized by hearing yelling and screaming. Many childhood abuse survivors report being hypersensitive to any loud or abusive discussion, whether it occurs among friends or on a television show.

- **Living in Perpetual Fear**

Growing up as the kid of an alcoholic or other abuser might leave you feeling fearful all of the time. Unfortunately, that dread might linger and be reactivated in the future by less serious situations.

This is how one person put it:

"Every day was a nightmare. Every day, I was afraid of what would happen when my father returned home. I was usually sweating profusely when I got home from school, praying that he wouldn't beat up on my mother or cause a ruckus. I was pondering what might happen when my father returned home. Is he going to be inebriated? Is he going to beat up on me or on my mother?"

There was a justification for perpetual worry if you grew up in a comparable environment. Despite this, many adult children keep this dread long after the source of the anxiety has passed.

- **Bullies find it easy to pick on you.**

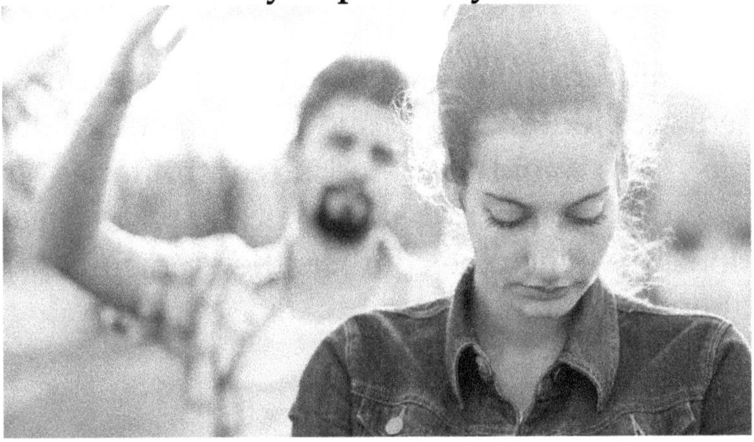

Bullies frequently target adult children who grew up with an alcoholic or toxic parent. Bullying in schools is well-known, but bullying within the home is also all too common.

We've all heard about how predators in the wild can "smell fear," and the same thing can happen to humans. It's almost as if an adult kid of an alcoholic appears weak or victimized, inviting individuals with a history of substance misuse or narcissistic qualities to abuse them.

Therapy or joining a support group can be quite beneficial in combating this behavior. You can role-play demonstrating confidence in interactions with others in the secure setting of an in-person or online support group. Forming trusted relationships can also help you reclaim control and reinforce a healthy adult relationship paradigm.

- **Conflict Avoidance Techniques**

Adult children of alcoholics and others who were abused as children are prone to conflict avoidance. People try to avoid any kind of confrontation, even the type of conflict that is necessary in healthy relationships, since the conflicts they remember from childhood are so unpleasant.

Underage Drinking Problem

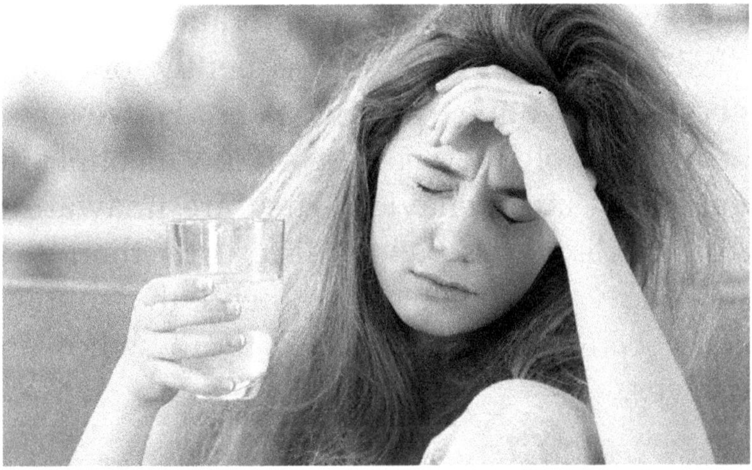

There are so many young individuals that drink. Alcohol is used by far more young people than tobacco or illegal narcotics. By the age of 18, more than 70% of teens have consumed at least one alcoholic drink.

When young individuals drink, they drink a large amount of alcohol at once. Teens drink less alcohol than adults. When teenagers do drink, though, they consume more alcohol than adults. On average, young people consume 5 drinks in one sitting. This is known as binge drinking, and it is an extremely risky manner of drinking that can result in significant issues and even death.

Early drinking can lead to alcohol later in life. Around 40% of those who began drinking before the age of 15 report they exhibit indications of alcohol. This is four times greater than the rate for those who did not start drinking until they were 21.

Young people may be particularly drawn to alcohol. Teenage years are a time of exploration, challenges, and risk-taking. Alcohol is frequently one of the dangers that young people face. However, the majority of people are unaware of how alcohol affects a teen's body and behavior. They are unaware that alcohol affects young people differently than it does adults. They also don't comprehend that underage drinkers can cause harm to those who aren't themselves.

Underage drinking can have serious consequences.

Many individuals are unaware that underage alcohol is a serious problem.

• Is a leading cause of injury-related death among young people.

Approximately 5,000 persons under the age of 21 die each year as a result of underage drinking; this includes roughly 1,900 deaths from car accidents, 1,600 deaths from homicides, 300 deaths from suicide, and hundreds more deaths from other injuries such as falls, burns, and drowning.

• Raises the chances of committing or being a victim of physical or sexual assault.

• Has a variety of effects on the body. Alcohol has a wide range of effects, from hangovers to death from alcohol poisoning.

• Can lead to a slew of other issues. Bad grades in school, run-ins with the authorities, and drug addiction are just a few examples.

• Affects a young person's ability to assess risk and make wise decisions. After drinking, an adolescent may believe there is nothing wrong with driving a car or travelling with a drunk driver.

• Is involved in dangerous sexual behaviour. This can lead to an increase in teen pregnancy and sexually transmitted illnesses (STDs), such as HIV, the AIDS-causing virus.

• Can be harmful to a developing brain, especially if teens drink excessive amounts of alcohol. We now know that the brain develops from infancy through adolescence and into the mid-twenties.

Teenage Years Are a Time of Many Transitions

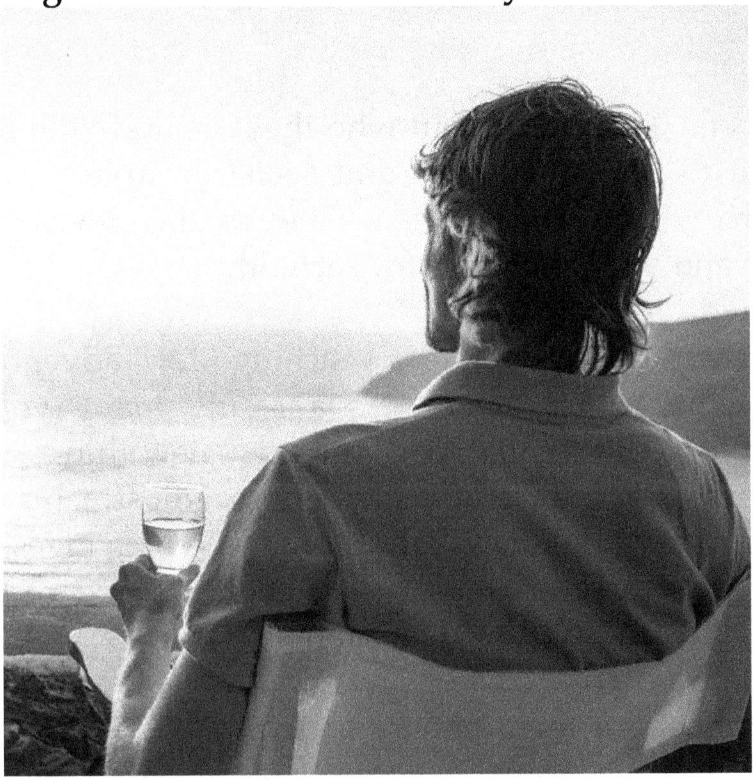

• Boys physically mature into young men, whereas girls mature into young ladies.

• Students progress from elementary to middle school to high school. Responsibilities increase as time goes on. Teens, for example, learn to drive, may acquire a job, and have more responsibilities and schoolwork than adults.

• Teenagers spend far less time with their parents. They prefer to spend time alone or with their buddies. They also prefer to sleep in and stay up later.

• Teens try to figure out who they are and who they want to be. Friendships and social groupings are a source of concern for them. They're also developing love and sexual feelings for each other.

• There is a greater yearning for adventure, excitement, and action. As a result, many young people desire to take more risks, try new things, and become more self-sufficient. These adjustments are crucial on the path to adulthood. These changes, on the other hand, enhance the likelihood that certain young people will turn to alcohol.

Why do some teens choose to drink?

The various "worlds" in which teens live can have a significant impact on their drinking. Some young individuals are more closely associated with their families than others. Others go to their friends for help first. Others seek for social groupings such as sports teams and clubs, faith-based organisations, or groups of like-minded young people. The Internet, media, music, and videos are also a big part of most youths' lives. All of these factors influence a young person's decision to consume alcohol.

Many factors influence a young person's decision to drink—

• The several "worlds" that teens inhabit, such as family, friends, school, and community

• A higher willingness to take risks, less dependence on parents, and increased independence

• Spending more time with friends and alone increases stress.

• They are more aware of what they see and hear about alcohol.

Even persons who do not drink can be affected by underage drinking.

• Drinking under the influence of alcohol while under the age of 21 can lead to risky behavior, property destruction, and violence.

• The drinker, as well as those in the vicinity, may suffer damage or even death as a result.

• People other than the driver make up about 45 percent of those killed in car accidents involving a drunk driver under the age of 21.

Everyone can feel the consequences of underage drinking. As a result, underage alcohol becomes an issue for everyone.

It is everyone's responsibility to put an end to underage drinking.

• Everyone can work together to build a community where young people can grow up without drinking and feel good about themselves.

• Everyone in the community should send the message that drinking while under the age of 21 is not acceptable. Whether youth hear the message at school, at home, at places of worship, on the sports field, in youth programmes, or in other areas where young people congregate, the message should be the same.

• Staying involved in their children's lives can assist avoid underage drinking. It is critical for families to be aware of what is going on with their teens.

• Young people can learn about the consequences of drinking too much alcohol. They have the power to affect how they and others view drinking.

What can local governments do to combat underage drinking?

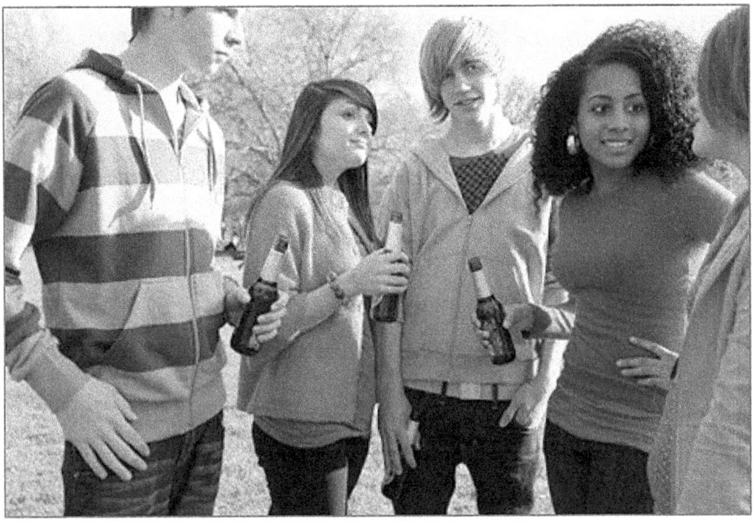

• When many teens drink, it is not a given that they will use alcohol while under the age of 21.

Change will require the participation of everyone in the community. We can all play a role in changing attitudes around teen drinking and helping to create conditions that prevent underage drinking. After all, changing people's minds is difficult. Adults are permitted to consume drinking. As a result, some individuals believe that drinking is a rite of passage for teenagers. Many young people believe that drinking makes them feel more mature. People of all ages forget that drinking while under the age of 21 is both unlawful and harmful. Communities can band together to promote a more positive attitude toward underage drinking. People's attitudes and behaviours can be influenced by a community that rejects underage drinking. However, it takes time. As a result, it's critical to keep communicating the message that underage drinking is unacceptable in the community. Communities can work together to support teen decisions not to drink.

Organize yourself.

- Address underage drinking as a public health and safety issue that everyone can help solve.
- Form groups to improve public perceptions of underage alcohol. Support the message that drinking under the age of 21 is not acceptable.
- Collaborate with community event sponsors to assist them deliver the message that underage drinking is not tolerated.

Knowledge should be shared.

- Spread the word about anti-underage drinking legislation. This includes age verification for persons purchasing alcohol over the internet.
- Assist people in learning about the most recent research on underage alcohol consumption. Include information for teens and others about the dangers of youth alcohol usage. Ending underage drinking requires a well-informed public.

Inform young people about the dangers of alcohol when under the age of 21. Support programs that assist teens who are already drinking.

Make a change in the teen scene.

Create welcoming, alcohol-free spaces for teens to congregate. Create programs that allow young people to grow, explore their options, prosper, and feel good about them without the use of alcohol, such as volunteer work. Encourage teens to recognize that, like "taking drugs" or smoking, underage drinking is harmful to their health and can have a negative influence on their lives. Encourage teens who are drinking under the influence to seek and accept help.

Make a move.

- Work to influence public perceptions of underage drinking. Put as much emphasis on underage drinking as on cigarette and drug usage in the community.

- Collaborate with state, tribal, and local organizations to combat underage drinking.

- Make it easier for young people who are drinking under the influence or who are at danger of doing so to get help.

- Disseminate information regarding underage drinking regulations. One of them is the law that makes drinking under the age of 21 unlawful. Other laws prohibit the sale or distribution of alcohol to minors. Others have made it illegal to drink and drive. Work to ensure that these laws are always followed.

Having a conversation with your child regarding alcohol use

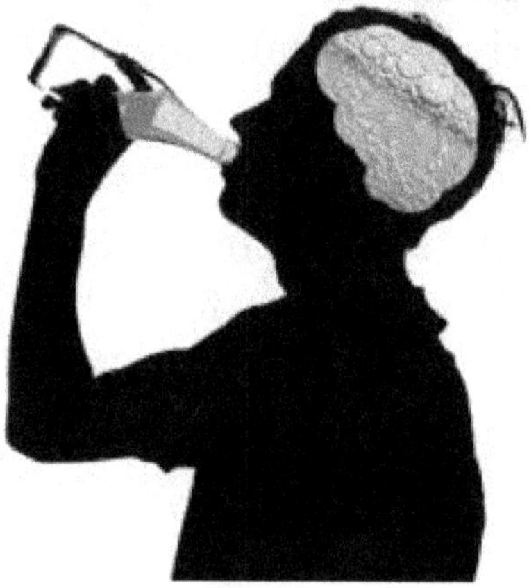

Talking to your child about alcohol use can be difficult, but it's a crucial part of preventing or limiting your child's alcohol use.

You may make unpleasant discussions easier by planning ahead of time what you want to say. You'll be ready if your child brings up the subject of alcohol consumption unexpectedly. You can also bring up the subject with your child before she inquires.

For instance, you may take discussions regarding alcohol as an opportunity to:

- Talk about your family's alcohol values and expectations.
- provide information about the effects of alcohol on the body, as well as how it impacts thinking and behavior.
- Describe the size of a regular drink, for example.

It's easier to bring up concerns like alcohol usage with your child when you have a close relationship with him, so make an effort to stay connected. And having open discussions about these topics allows you to learn more about what's going on in your child's life. As a result, you'll be in a better position to assist him in dealing with challenging situations as they arise.

Drinking's Effects on Your Body

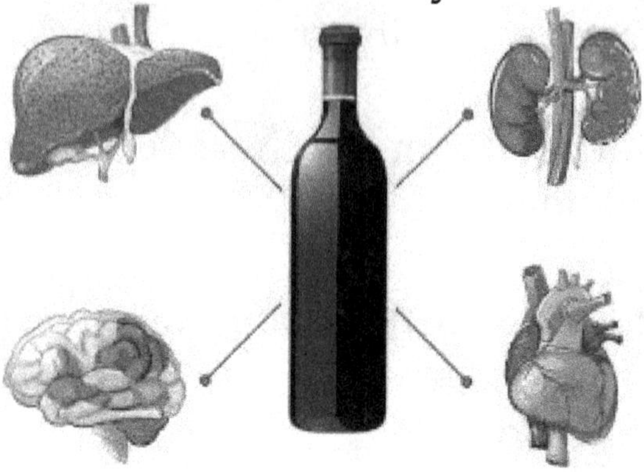

The effects of alcohol on your body begin the moment you take your first sip. While a glass of wine with dinner isn't harmful in and of itself, the long-term effects of drinking wine, beer, or spirits can be detrimental.

A glass of wine a day could be beneficial to your overall health. However, if the habit develops or if you find it difficult to stop after just one glass, the cumulative effects can be significant.

- **Endocrine and digestive glands**

Drinking too much alcohol might cause the pancreas' digestive enzymes to become activated abnormally. The buildup of these enzymes can cause pancreatitis, or inflammation of the pancreas. Pancreatitis can develop into a long-term illness with dangerous consequences.

- **Damage caused by inflammation**

The liver is an organ that helps your body break down and remove toxic substances, such as alcohol. This process is hampered by long-term alcohol consumption. It also raises your chances of developing chronic liver inflammation and illness. Cirrhosis is the scarring caused by this inflammation. The liver is destroyed by the creation of scar tissue. The liver has a tougher time eliminating poisonous compounds from your body as it grows more impaired.

Liver illness is life-threatening and causes a buildup of poisons and waste in the body. Women are more likely than men to acquire alcoholic liver disease. Women's bodies are more prone to absorbing more alcohol and processing it for longer periods of time. Women also show signs of liver disease sooner than males.

Liver Disease Caused by Alcohol

Overview

Damage to the liver from years of excessive drinking causes alcohol-related liver disease (ARLD). Alcohol misuse can cause the liver to swell and become inflamed over time. Cirrhosis is a scarring condition caused by liver injury. Cirrhosis is the most advanced form of liver disease.

ARLD is a significant public health issue. Approximately 8% to 10% of Americans drink excessive amounts of alcohol. Ten to fifteen percent of people will develop ARLD. Women who drink more than eight alcoholic beverages per week are categorised as heavy drinkers, while males who drink more than 15 are labelled as drinking drinkers.

Excessive alcohol use has a number of negative repercussions, including liver damage. This is particularly dangerous because liver failure is deadly. Learn how to avoid and manage this life-threatening disease.

Types of alcohol-related liver disease and its symptoms

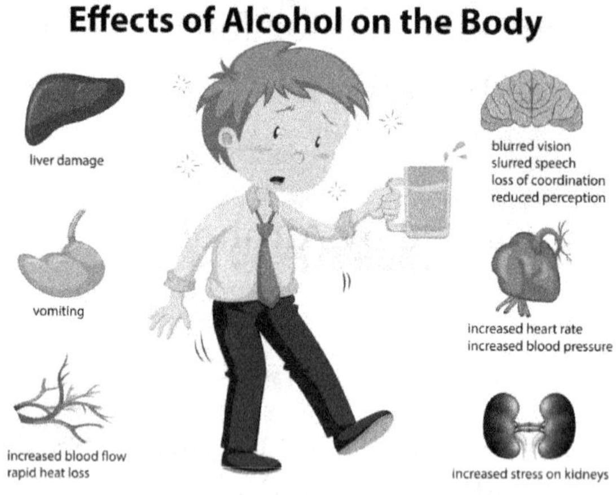

The symptoms of ARLD vary depending on where the disease is in its progression. There are three stages to the process:

Fatty liver disease caused by alcoholism:

The first stage of ARLD is when fat begins to build up around the liver. It can be healed by refraining from drinking alcohol.

Acute alcoholic hepatitis (AAH) is a type of alcoholic hepatitis that occurs

In this stage, alcohol consumption promotes liver inflammation (swelling). The outcome is determined by the extent of the injury. Treatment may be able to restore the damage in some situations, but more severe cases of alcoholic hepatitis can result in liver failure.

Cirrhosis due to alcoholism:

ARLD in this kind is the most severe. The liver has been harmed by alcohol addiction at this point, and the damage cannot be reversed. Cirrhosis is a condition that can result in liver failure.

Some patients with ARLD do not have symptoms until the disease has progressed. Others begin to show symptoms early. ARLD symptoms include:

- nausea
- a decrease in appetite

- jaundice
- fatigue
- Anxiety in the stomach
- an increase in thirst
- swollen legs and abdomen
- Loss of weight
- Skin pigmentation (darkening or lightening)
- hands or feet that are red
- bowel motions that are dark
- fainting
- agitation that is unusual
- mood changes
- confusion
- Gums that leak
- Breast enlargement (in men)

After binge drinking, ARLD symptoms may appear more frequently.

Alcohol-related liver disease risk factors

If you have any of the following conditions, you're more likely to develop ARLD:

If you have a history of ARLD in your family

- You frequently drink a large amount of alcohol
- you are a binge drinker
- You are malnourished.

Acute alcoholic hepatitis can also be caused by binge drinking. This is potentially fatal. Acute alcoholic hepatitis can develop in women after four drinks and in men after five drinks.

Alcohol-related liver disease diagnosis

ARLD isn't the only condition that can harm the liver. To rule out other disorders, your doctor will want to assess the health of your liver. Your doctor may issue the following orders:

- a full blood count (CBC)
- A liver function test is performed.
- a computed tomography (CT) scan of the abdomen
- Ultrasound of the abdomen
- a biopsy of the liver

The liver function test also includes liver enzyme testing. Three liver enzymes are measured in these tests:

- Glutamyltransferase (gamma-glutamyltransferase) (GGT)
- aspartate aminotransferase (aspartate aminotransferase) (AST)
- alanine aminotransferase is a protein that converts alanine to alanine (ALT)

If your AST level is two times higher than your ALT level, you're likely to have ARLD. This finding is found in approximately 80% of ARLD patients, according to the National Institute on Alcohol Abuse and Alcoholism.

Taking care of alcoholic liver illness

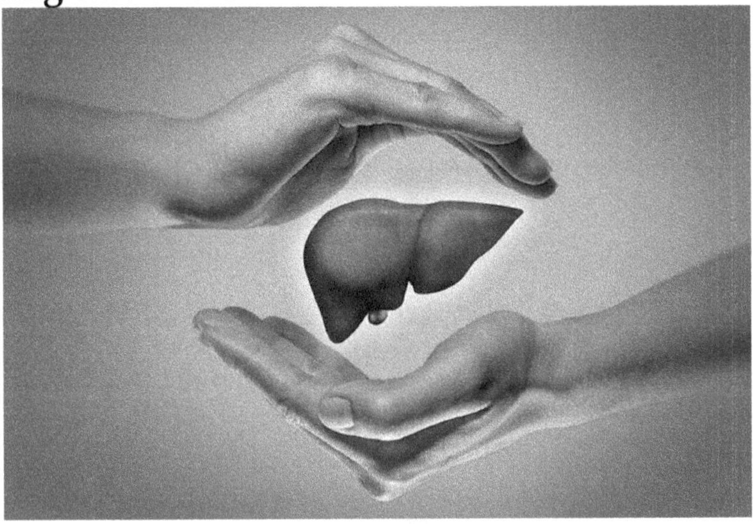

The treatment of ARLD involves two objectives. The first is to assist you in quitting drinking. This can help mend the liver and prevent additional damage. The second step is to improve the health of your liver.

If you have ARLD, your doctor may suggest that you do the following:

Alcoholic rehabilitation programmes, such as Alcoholics Anonymous, can assist you in quitting drinking if you are unable to do it on your own.

Multivitamins: People who drink a lot of alcohol have a deficiency in B-complex vitamins. Anemia or malnutrition can result from this deficit.

If your liver is too scarred by cirrhosis to function correctly, you may need a liver transplant.

Vitamin A supplements: Vitamin A deficiency is common in persons with ARLD.

It's vital to remember that combining vitamin A and alcohol can be fatal. These vitamins are only for persons who have given up drinking. Supplements won't heal your liver condition, but they can help you avoid problems like malnutrition.

Alcohol-related liver disease complications

ARLD complications can include:

- persistent scarring and loss of function in the liver
- esophageal varies that hemorrhage (enlarged veins in the esophagus that develop in people who have liver disease)
- increased blood pressure in the liver's blood vessels (portal hypertension)
- Toxin accumulation in the blood causes a loss of brain function (hepatic encephalopathy)

- **Blood sugar levels**

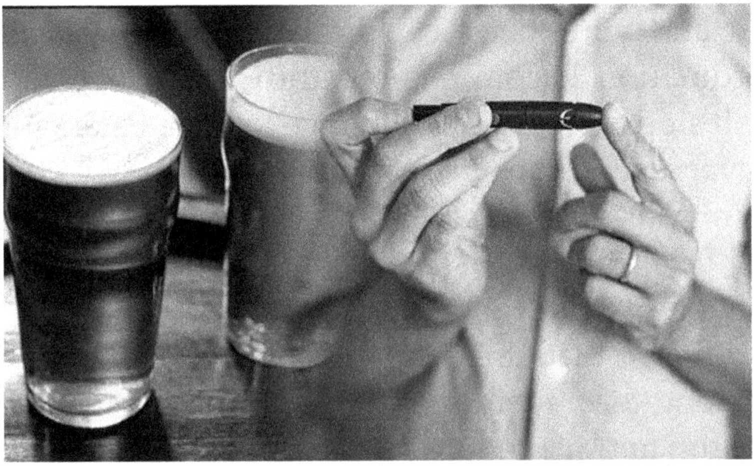

The pancreas aids in the regulation of insulin utilization and glucose response in the body. When your pancreas and liver aren't working properly, you face the danger of hypoglycemia, or low blood sugar. A malfunctioning pancreas may also make it difficult for the body to produce enough insulin to use sugar. Hyperglycemia, or an excess of sugar in the blood, can result.

You may face more difficulties and side effects from diabetes if your body is unable to manage and balance your blood sugar levels. Excessive alcohol consumption should be avoided by those with diabetes or hypoglycemia.

- **Central nervous system**

Understanding how alcohol affects your central nervous system is one of the simplest ways to comprehend its effects on your body. One of the first indicators that you've had too much to drink is slurred speech. The communication between your

brain and your body can be hampered by alcohol. Coordination becomes more difficult as a result of this. It's possible that you'll have trouble balancing. It is never a good idea to drive after drinking.
You may have numbness and tingling sensations in your feet and hands as alcohol causes additional harm to your central nervous system.
In addition, drinking impairs your brain's ability to form long-term memories. It also impairs your ability to reason and make sensible decisions. Damage to the frontal lobe can occur over time. This part of the brain is in charge of emotional regulation, short-term memory, and judgment, among other things.

Alcohol addiction that is both chronic and severe might result in lasting brain damage. This can develop to Wernicke-Korsakoff syndrome, a memory-related brain condition.

- **Dependency**

Some persons who drink a lot of alcohol may develop a physical and emotional dependence on it. Withdrawing from alcohol can be both difficult and dangerous. When it comes to overcoming an alcohol addiction, professional assistance is frequently required. As a result, many people seek medical detoxification in order to recover from their addiction. It's the safest technique to ensure you don't develop a physical dependency. Detoxification can be done as an outpatient or as an inpatient, depending on the danger of withdrawal symptoms.

The following are some of the signs and symptoms of alcohol withdrawal:

- anxiety
- nervousness
- nausea
- tremors
- hypertension (high blood pressure)
- unsteady heartbeat
- excessive sweating

Seizures, hallucinations, and delirium are all possible side effects of severe withdrawal.

- The digestive tract

The link between alcohol intake and your digestive system may not be obvious at first. Often, the side effects do not manifest until after the damage has occurred. And the more you drink, the worse the consequences will be.

Drinking can harm your digestive tract tissues, making it difficult for your intestines to digest food and absorb nutrients and vitamins. Malnutrition may arise as a result.

Heavy drinking can also lead to the following:

- gassiness
- bloating
- a feeling of bloating in your stomach
- constipation or diarrhea

Ulcers or hemorrhoids (related to dehydration and constipation) are not uncommon in heavy drinkers. They also have the potential to induce serious internal bleeding. If ulcers are not recognized and treated promptly, they can be fatal.

Overconsumption of alcohol may put people at risk for cancer. People who drink alcohol on a regular basis are more prone to develop cancers of the mouth, throat, esophagus, colon, or liver. People who drink and smoke on a regular basis are at an even higher risk of cancer.

System of circulation

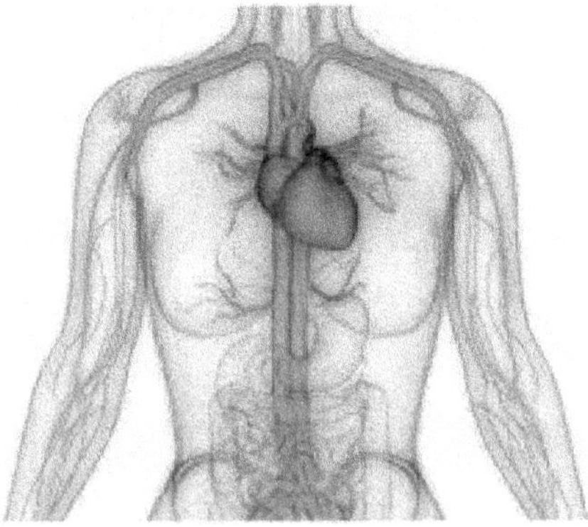

Alcohol can have a negative impact on your heart and lungs. People who drink alcohol on a regular basis have a higher risk of heart disease than those who do not. Women who drink are more prone than men to acquire heart disease.

Complications of the circulatory system include:

- hypertension (high blood pressure)
- unsteady heartbeat
- inability to circulate blood throughout the body
- stroke
- cardiac arrest
- Cardiovascular disease
- a heart attack

Anemia is caused by a lack of ability to absorb vitamins and minerals from meals. This is a condition in which your red blood cell count is low. Fatigue is one of the most common symptoms of anaemia.

Sexual and reproductive health is both important.

You may believe that drinking alcohol will help you have more fun in bed by lowering your inhibitions. The truth, however, is considerably different. Erectile dysfunction is more common in men who drink excessively. Heavy drinking can also lower your libido and impede the generation of sex hormones.

Women who drink excessive amounts of alcohol may experience a cessation of menstruation. As a result, they are at a higher risk of infertility. Premature birth, miscarriage, and stillbirth are all risks for women who drink extensively during pregnancy.

Women who drink alcohol while pregnant endanger their unborn kid. FASDs (foetal alcohol syndrome disorders) are a severe problem. There are also the following conditions:

- difficulty in learning
- health problems that have been present for a long time
- an increase in emotional issues
- anomalies in physical development

Muscle and skeletal systems
Long-term alcohol consumption may impair your body's ability to maintain bone strength. Thinner bones and a higher risk of fractures if you fall as a

result of this behavior. Fractures may also take longer to heal.

Alcohol use can cause muscle weakening, cramps, and finally atrophy.

Immune system (Immune system)

Your body's natural immune system is weakened by heavy drinking. It becomes more difficult for your body to fight off invading germs and viruses as a result of this.

People who drink heavily for a long time are also more prone than the average population to get pneumonia or tuberculosis. Alcohol intake is linked to about 10% of all TB cases worldwide. Drinking alcohol also raises your chances of developing cancers of the mouth, breast, and colon.

Quitting alcohol

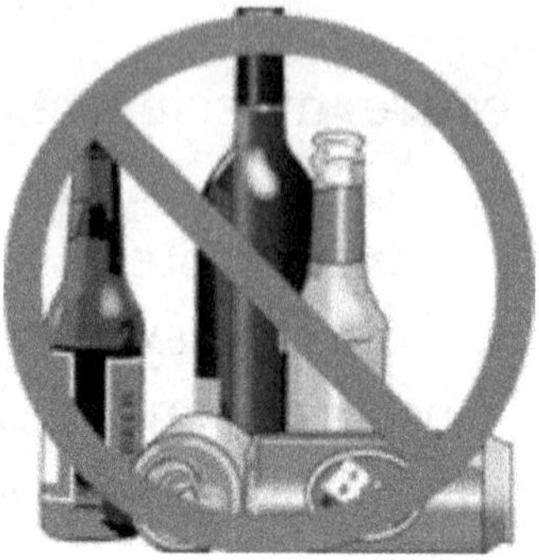

Drinking is widely regarded as a social pastime, a stress reliever, and even a potential treatment for insomnia and anxiety.

However, alcohol rarely helps to alleviate these problems in the long run. It does, however, have some substantial drawbacks.

Even modest drinking can make you feel drowsy, foggy, or hungover. The more you drink, the more probable you are to have various negative health impacts, such as:

- sleep disturbances
- gastrointestinal problems
- issues with memory

- Anxiety, depression, and irritability are all on the rise.

- quarrels and various forms of strife with family and friends

You might start to question if it's time to take a break when these consequences start to build up. And you're not the only one who feels this way. More and more people are examining the role alcohol plays in their lives, from monthlong sobriety challenges to the #SoberCurious campaign.

These guidelines will help you design a strategy that works for you, whether you're wanting to cut back or take an indefinite hiatus.

Take some time to think about your relationship with alcohol first.

Identifying why you're doing something is a crucial first step in giving up anything.

- **Calculate how much you drink on a regular basis.**

Maybe you don't think you're addicted to alcohol, but you still question whether you're drinking too much.

When you go without drinking, say you don't get any cravings. Nonetheless, "a quick drink" frequently turns into three or four. When you're having a wonderful time, it's difficult to quit, especially when you're among pals who are having the same kind of fun.

- **Consider why you drink.**

Perhaps your issues are more about your reasons for drinking than the amount. Many people use alcohol to numb emotional anguish or make it easier to deal with difficult situations. On a first date or before a difficult conversation, it's usual to drink to de-stress.

However, if facing issues without alcohol is difficult, it's worth evaluating whether drinking stops you from developing more effective coping mechanisms.

Cyndi Turner, LCSW, LSATP, MAC, a Virginia therapist who specialises in addiction therapy and alcohol moderation, says knowing why you drink is crucial.

She goes on to say that understanding the causes for your alcohol – whether it's because of relationship stress, work problems, insomnia, or something else – can help you find more effective methods to deal with those challenges.

- **Justifications for abstaining from drinking alcoholic beverages**

Alcoholism is recognised to create a variety of health, mental, and social issues. Alcoholism can cause liver disease such as cirrhosis, which occurs when good tissue is replaced with scar tissue and the liver is unable to function normally. Your kidneys are in jeopardy, and there's a good chance you'll develop anxiety issues as a result. Alcohol has a lot of calories. Most drinkers will frequently drink alcohol during a meal. The body will be starved and willing to eat everything. Typically, at 2 a.m., you'll find yourself snacking on some fairly unhealthy items just to keep yourself awake. As a result, alcohol has the potential to contribute to obesity.

- **Think about your strategy.**

You may be aware that you desire to completely abstain from using alcohol. However, you may be unsure about stopping totally and don't want to commit to that objective.

That's perfectly OK. The most essential thing is to examine your drinking patterns and come up with a plan that works for you.

Without total sobriety, it is possible to improve one's relationship with alcohol and make more thoughtful, educated drinking decisions.

Turner's method to moderation management is just one of many alternatives to complete sobriety.

It emphasises choosing the best approach for your situation, not someone else's, in order to reduce alcohol usage and the associated consequences that come with it.

Of course, complete sobriety is a good goal, but it doesn't have to be the only one.

Don't know what you want to achieve yet? That's fine as well. Just keep in mind that you have options.

Let's talk about it.

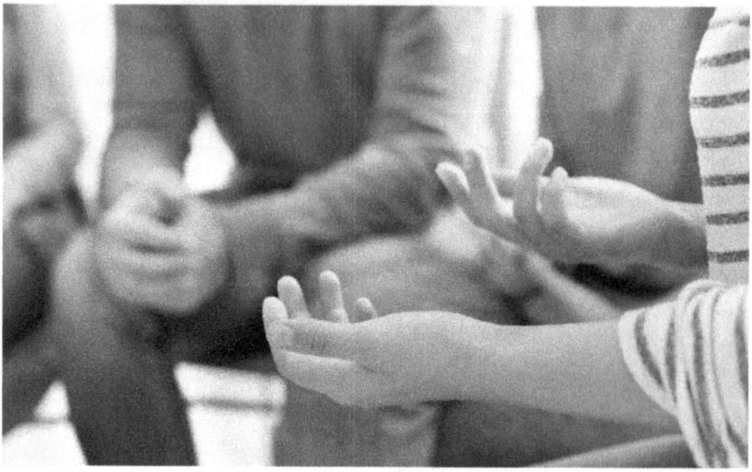

Allowing others to know about your decision to stop drinking may encourage you to keep with it.

- **Involve your family and friends.**

When you stop drinking, your family and friends can offer you encouragement and support.

You might persuade people to examine their own drinking habits if you open up about your relationship with alcohol.

Perhaps your partner, sibling, or roommate is considering a shift as well. You may support one other while also increasing your drive and accountability by changing your drinking habits together.

Turner emphasizes the necessity of having a trustworthy support person with you when attending alcohol-related events. When you don't have to do it alone, it's much easier to say no to a drink.

- **Look for a group to join.**

Developing new ties with folks who abstain from alcohol can be quite beneficial.

Turner adds, "The more support you have, the better."

Here are some suggestions:

Why not invite a different coworker to check out the new bakery down the block instead of putting your commitment to the test by joining your coworkers for happy hour?

Consider forming friendships and romantic relationships with people who do not regard drinking as a significant part of their lives.

Do you miss the buzz of a bar? You might be possible to go to a sober bar and socialize without drinking depending on where you reside.

To locate other people interested in alcohol-free activities, use applications like Meet up.

- **Know what you're going to say**

People may wonder why you decline a drink.

You're not compelled to provide specifics, but having a ready response can help:

“I'm reducing my consumption to improve my health.”

“I don't like how I feel after drinking.”

You don't have to say anything more than "No, thank you." When you practice your rejection ahead of time, you will feel more at ease and confident when you are confronted with an alcohol-related circumstance.

Don't be concerned about others judging you; the majority of people are unlikely to notice or remember what you do.

If you want to give a more detailed explanation to loved ones but aren't sure what to say, make your explanation simple:

“I've been drinking excessively for no apparent reason, and I'd like to spend some time reconsidering that habit.”

"I see that I drink when I don't want to face my feelings, and I want to improve my ability to go through them without the need of alcohol."

"I don't enjoy drinking, and I'm tired of doing it only to please others."

- **Alter your surroundings**

Drinking can become a natural response when alcohol is a part of your daily routine, especially when you are anxious or overwhelmed.

To stop drinking, you may not need to fully overhaul your life, but a few modifications in your environment can make a tremendous difference.

- **Quit drinking alcohol.**

When you're attempting to quit smoking, having alcohol in your home can be tempting. If you're in the mood for a drink, knowing you'll have to go out and get anything can keep you distracted long enough to find something else to do.

Maintain a supply of nonalcoholic beverages for yourself and others. To be a good host, you don't have to serve alcohol. Allow guests to bring their own alcohol, which they can keep and take with them when they leave.

If you share a room with roommates, ask them to keep their alcohol hidden rather than in common areas.

Discover a new favourite drink.

Choosing the correct substitute beverage will help you stay committed to your goal of quitting drinking. Although plain water has numerous health benefits, it is admittedly not the most exciting option.

You may find something fun that doesn't make you miss your favourite drink with a little creativity.

Try:

- adding chopped fruits or herbs to plain or sparkling water
- infusing tea, apple cider, or hot chocolate with cinnamon sticks or spices
- grape juice or lemonade mixed with sparkling water

Grapes are one of the most common and well-known methods for overcoming alcohol addiction. If you're craving a drink of alcoholic alcohol, all things being equal, have a glass of grape juice or eat a lot of grapes. Grapes are an exceptional alternative for heavy drinkers because they are the source from which wine is manufactured. Furthermore, these natural items are high in potassium, which helps your body maintain a healthy blood balance while also energising the kidneys. Grapes can also effectively remove toxins from the liver.

Juices from fruits

This conventional remedy appears to be effective for some people. If you're a heavy alcohol, you'll need to add new, custom-made juices to your diet to kick the habit. These juices are high in vitamin A, folate, vitamin C, calcium, magnesium, and potassium, and can be consumed at any time.

Juice from dates

If you're trying to break free from alcohol, go on dates on a regular basis. These organic ingredients offer qualities that aid in detoxification and the removal of toxins from your liver. After soaking a few dates in water for an hour, remove the seeds and smash them in the water. To have the best results, drink this beverage twice a day for a long time.

Gourd Juice is a bitter drink made from gourds.

Severe gourd heals liver damage caused with excessive alcohol consumption. This vegetable is a well-known treatment for flushing toxins from the body. To make the drink, squeeze the juice from a couple of severe gourd leaves into a glass of buttermilk and combine 3 tsp. To free yourself from alcohol servitude, drink the mixture on an empty stomach for a few months.

Juice of carrots

Carrots are also one of the most popular ingredients for reducing the desire to drink alcohol. This is due to carrots' multiple medical benefits and supplements, as well as their nutritional value. Simply drink a glass of carrot juice whenever you feel the want to consume alcohol. Because it improves processing and relieves alcohol fixation, you will feel better. To get rid of your alcohol cravings, drink a glass of carrot juice every day.

Change up your routine.

When you have a habit of drinking at a certain time of day, one of the greatest ways to break the pattern is to do something else. The most beneficial activities are those that get you out of the house and moving.

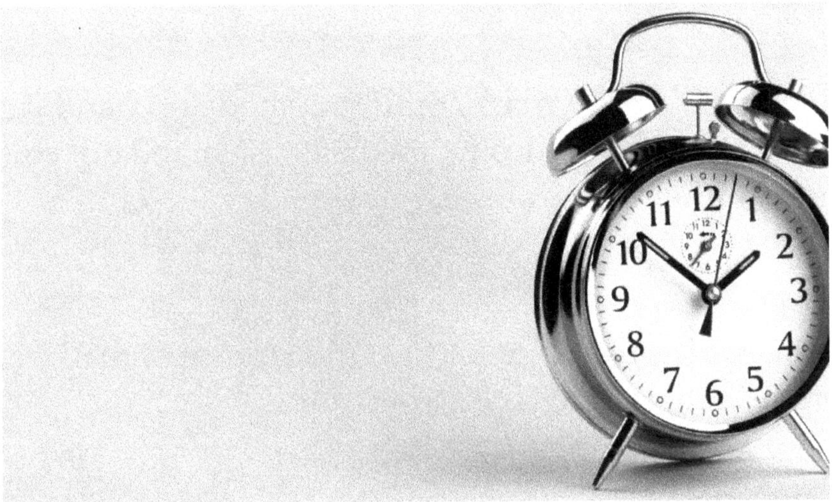

Consider the following suggestions:

If you regularly meet pals for a drink after work, take a stroll with them or meet them for a hangout in a park or other alcohol-free location.

Why not try a new spot that doesn't serve alcohol instead of your typical restaurant for dinner and drinks? You'll be able to do something else without feeling compelled to drink.

Make it a habit to cook at home to keep yourself occupied and save money.

Having a few alternate coping methods on hand can assist when your desire to drink is linked to your mood rather than a specific time of day:

Instead of a drink, try affirmations, deep breathing, or meditation to relieve anxiety.

Reach out to a loved one or watch a favourite movie when you're feeling lonely.

Make time for yourself.

It can be really distressing to stop drinking. When you use alcohol to cope with emotional discomfort, the added overwhelm can trigger the need to drink, making success much more elusive.

When making major changes, it's natural to feel overwhelmed, but basic self-care habits can help you manage your emotions and take care of your mind and body.

Make health a top priority.

Physical well-being can help you cope with circumstances that trigger the need to drink by increasing your resilience and emotional strength.

You're taking a significant step toward bettering your physical health by avoiding alcohol. You'll likely feel more invigorated and motivated to continue your progress as you realise the health benefits.

Other things to think about:

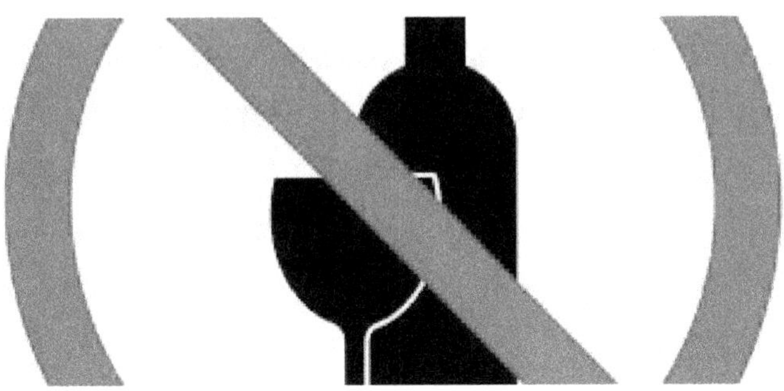

Keep yourself hydrated.

Eat well-balanced meals on a regular basis. Include foods that will give you more energy and improve your mood.

If you're able, engage in frequent physical activity. For fun activities to stay active, try hiking, cycling, dancing, or roller-skating.

Make getting a better night's sleep a priority. Most individuals should aim for 7 to 9 hours of sleep.

Rekindle old passions

To deal with boredom, many people turn to alcohol. Satisfying hobbies not only keep you from drinking, but they also help you relax, which is something everyone needs.

If you've lately discovered a desire to rekindle an old pastime, now is the time to do it.

You could try:

DIY home improvement projects

- constructing or painting models
- board games and video games
- volunteering
- relaxing with a good book

Keep a diary.

Maybe you've never been interested in writing down your innermost thoughts, but journaling can be a useful tool for keeping track of your emotions as you strive to quit alcohol.

Exploring what you find difficult and when you want to drink the most in writing can help you spot trends that provide greater insight into your alcohol usage.

Comparing the sensations you have when you drink to the feelings you have when you don't helps you identify when drinking doesn't solve the problems you're attempting to solve.

A journal can also be used to write down reasons for quitting and develop activities to replace drinking.

Investigate novel coping mechanisms.

Once you've figured out some of the key reasons why you drink, you may start looking for alternative ways to deal with those triggers.

The most effective coping method is often determined by the situation:

When you're upset but need some alone time, consider listening to a favourite record or reading a reassuring book.

You might vent to a loved one or practise improved communication skills to reconnect with your partner if you want to drink to avoid relationship problems or stress.

If loneliness makes you want to drink, consider finding ways to connect with long-distance friends or forming new friendships.

Getting Rid of Alcoholism

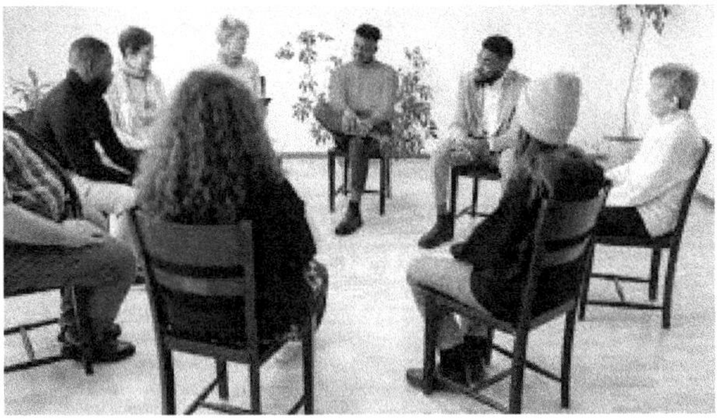

What's the best way for me to quit drinking?

Overcoming an alcohol addiction can be a long and winding road. It may even seem impossible at times. However, this is not the case. You can recover from alcoholism and alcohol abuse, no matter how intense your drinking or how powerless you feel, if you're ready to quit drinking and willing to seek the help you need. You don't have to wait until you've struck rock bottom to make a change; you may start now. These tips will help you get started on the path to recovery today, whether you want to stop drinking altogether or cut back to healthier levels.

The majority of persons who have alcohol problems do not decide to make a drastic shift or modify their drinking habits overnight. The process of recovery is usually more gradual. Denial is a major roadblock in the early phases of change. You may make excuses and drag your feet even after acknowledging you have a drinking problem. It's critical to admit your reservations about quitting drinking. If you're not sure if you're ready to change or if you're having trouble deciding, consider the costs and benefits of each option.

Set objectives and plan for change.

- **How will you achieve your objectives?**

Write down some thoughts on how you may help yourself achieve your goals after you've set your goals to either stop or cut back on your drinking. Consider the following scenario:

Remove all temptations. Remove any alcoholic beverages, barware, and other similar items from your home and business.

- **Make your aim public.**

Tell your friends, family, and coworkers that you're attempting to quit or reduce your drinking. If they drink, urge them to refrain from doing so in front of you to help you recuperate.

Be honest with yourself about your new limitations. Make it clear that drinking is not permitted in your house, and that you may be unable to attend activities that serve alcohol.

- **Stay away from negative influences.**

Keep your distance from folks who don't support your efforts to quit drinking or who don't respect the boundaries you've established. It's possible that you'll have to say goodbye to certain acquaintances and social contacts as a result of this.

- **Take notes from the past.**

Consider your prior attempts to quit or cut down on your drinking. What worked for you? What didn't work? What can you do differently this time to prevent falling into the same traps as before?

Cutting back on alcohol vs. going completely

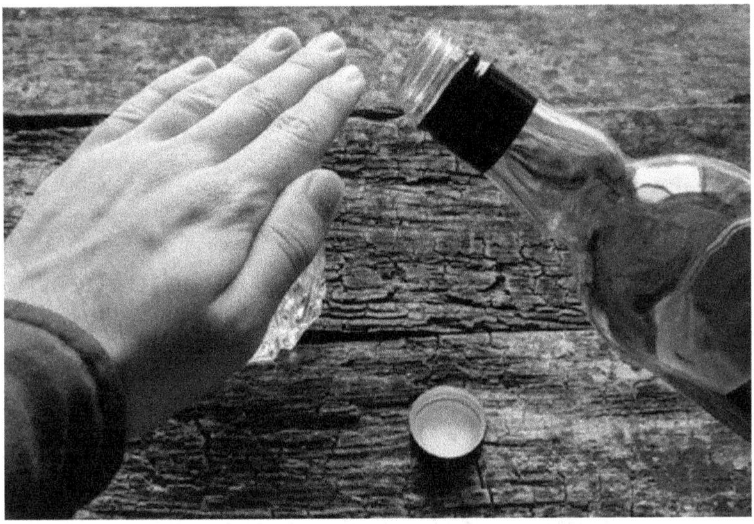

The degree of your drinking issue will determine whether or not you can successfully cut back on your drinking. It's better to try to stop drinking totally if you're an alcoholic, which means you can't regulate your drinking by definition. However, if you aren't ready to take that step, or if you don't have an alcohol addiction problem but wish to cut back for personal or health reasons, the following suggestions may be useful:

- **Decide on a drinking goal**

Choose a limit for how much you'll drink—no more than one drink per day if you're a woman, two drinks per day if you're a man—and set out some days each week when you won't drink any alcohol at all. Make a note of your drinking goal and keep it somewhere visible, such as on your phone or taped to your refrigerator.

- **Keep track of your drinking in order to meet your objective.**

Write down every time you have a drink and how much you drink for 3 to 4 weeks. You might be startled by your weekly drinking habits after reviewing the results.

- **Limit your drinking at home.**

Limit or eliminate alcohol from your home. If you don't have temptations around, it's much easier to resist drinking.

- **Take your time drinking.**

When you drink, take little sips and wait 30 minutes or an hour between drinks. Between alcoholic drinks, drink soda, water, or juice. It's never a good idea to drink on an empty stomach, so make sure you eat before you drink.

- **Each week, set aside one or two alcohol-free days.**

Then try to go a week without drinking. Make a mental and physical note of how you're feeling these days; noting the rewards may help you quit for good.

Treatment options for alcoholism

Some people can quit drinking on their own or with the assistance of a 12-step programme or another support group (see below for links). Others require medical care in order to safely and pleasantly abstain from alcohol. The best alternative for you is determined by how much you've been drinking, how long you've had a problem, the stability of your living circumstances, and any other health problems you may have.

Often, the initial step is to see your primary care physician, sometimes known as a GP. Your doctor can assess your drinking habits, diagnose any co-occurring problems, evaluate your overall health, and recommend you to therapy. They may be able to prescribe medicine to assist you in quitting.

5 WAYS STOP DRINKING HAS AN EFFECT ON YOUR BRAIN

Heavy alcohol use has well-known physical repercussions, such as liver damage and high blood pressure. However, any level of alcohol consumption is harmful to the brain.

Mental fog, anxiety, and mood swings can affect even moderate drinkers or those who have been drinking excessively for a short amount of time.

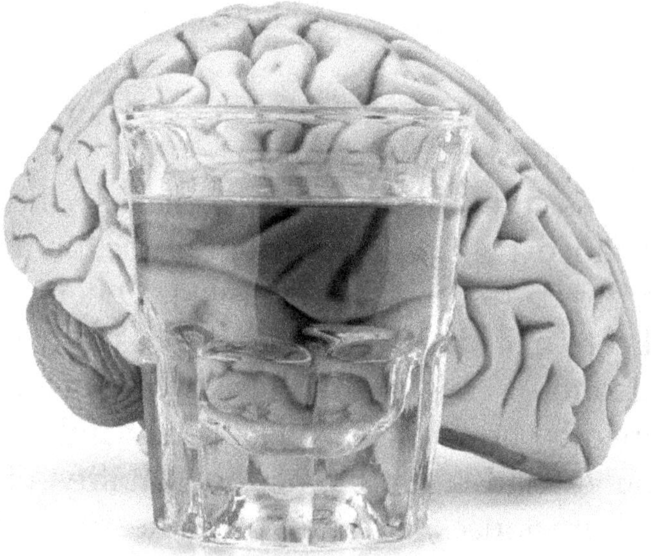

Brain changes impacting cognitive function and mood can become severe and debilitating in those who have an alcohol use disorder, binge drink, or have been drinking for a long time.

The good news is that simply abstaining from alcohol, even individuals who have spent years putting their brains off balance can begin to mend and restore its natural function. Here are some of the changes in your brain that will occur if you stop drinking.

- **Frontal lobe regeneration is a term used to describe the process of regenerating the frontal lob**

When you drink too much, the frontal lobe of the brain, which is responsible for several important activities like cognition, behaviour control, memory, and motor function, takes a beating.

Years of alcohol misuse can cause substantial damage to this part of the brain, resulting in a range of problems such as memory loss and the inability to think sensibly.

While patients in early recovery may still have these symptoms, as well as a difficulty to comprehend vast amounts of information, as time passes, new cell growth will begin to repair the damage.

In order to overcome addiction, rational decision-making and impulse control are essential, and happily, these brain processes will return as you heal.

- **Dopamine Levels Begin to Return to Normal**

Alcohol causes a complicated dopamine imbalance in the brain.

Dopamine is released when you engage in pleasurable activities, such as eating chocolate or participating in sports, and it teaches your brain which acts to repeat and eventually crave.

Alcohol causes the brain to become overloaded with dopamine while also lowering the number of dopamine receptors in the brain. The lack of dopamine and decreased receptors when you first stop drinking can make you feel melancholy and hopeless.

Excessively high or abnormally low levels of dopamine can have negative consequences, but without the use of alcohol, your brain will gradually adjust dopamine levels and responsiveness to the chemical.

- **The Return of Motivation**

As previously stated, early recovery may cause you to struggle with your mood and overall mental health, but as your body and brain improve, you will have renewed enthusiasm to develop healthy habits in your life.

This means you'll be able to engage in new activities, such as daily exercise, that will improve your mood and encourage brain cell growth.

For anyone recovering from addiction, the early days of abstinence can be tiring and stressful, but a balanced and healthy brain will return, along with a sense of heightened desire toward positive goals.

- **Increased Serotonin Production**

While alcohol has a short-term effect of increasing serotonin, a chemical that improves emotions of happiness and wellness, heavy alcohol usage often leads to a drop in serotonin levels, which increases the risk of depression.

Serotonin production might return to normal once you stop drinking. If you still have depression symptoms after you've recovered, you may need medication.

You can better understand your mental health and identify what you need to feel your best by removing alcohol from the equation.

- **As You Gain New Skills, Healthy Activity Returns**

Alcohol becomes a crutch for many chronic drinkers to cope with a variety of situations and emotions in daily life. You may have used alcohol to boost your confidence, handle stress, or fight depression.

While alcohol isn't a panacea for any of these issues, it can dull your natural reaction to life's events, making it difficult to operate without it. While early sobriety might be difficult, adjusting to life without alcohol necessitates the development of new coping strategies and social skills.

This is an opportunity for your brain power to expand and evolve when you resume your previous activities while sober.

Depending on how long you've been a heavy drinker, you might be socialising and regulating your emotions for the first time now that you're clean.

Your brain establishes new connections and pathways for future healthy interactions with the acquisition of each new coping skill and the progression of emotional maturity.

While the harm that heavy alcohol use may cause to your brain is alarming, it is fully possible to recover from addiction and begin to heal from the inside out.

7 Meditations to Help You Quit Drinking and Beat Alcoholism

Did you know that meditation can help you quit drinking?

According to a study published in the International Journal of Neuropsychopharmacology, just 11 minutes of mindfulness training followed by a continuing attempt to be aware can help alcoholics drink 9.3 units less each week on average.

Meditation is the nonjudgmental practise of focussing one's thoughts on the present moment. Breathing techniques, mantras, and guided meditations are all examples of meditation.

I'll show you how to stop drinking with meditation for alcoholism in this guide. I'll give you the science, my personal experiences, and my favourite exercises so you can stop drinking right now.

The Best Meditation Techniques for drinking Alcohol Today

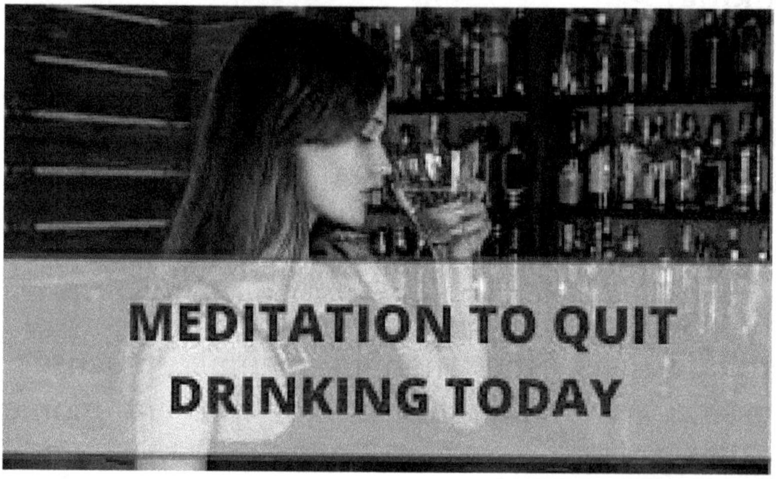

- **Meditation Script for "Quit Drinking"**

The screenplay that follows is designed to help you develop the ideal mindset for overcoming alcoholism. You will increase your mindfulness and develop forgiveness and self-compassion as a result of doing so.

1. Sit in a comfortable position with good posture. I recommend that you sit in a chair. Your feet should be shoulder-width apart. Make sure your knees are not locked and are comfortable. Rest your bottom on the seat so that your weight is equally distributed. Lengthen your spine by a few inches. To lengthen your neck,

tuck your chin down somewhat. Now turn your head 45 degrees forward, so you're gazing slightly downwards (slightly!).

2. Make the Gyan mudra with your hand (a mudra is a hand gesture). Place your hands on your thighs, palms facing upwards, to do this. Outwardly rest your third, fourth, and fifth fingers. Bring the tips of your thumbs and index fingers together in a fist. This position will assist you in concentrating.

3. Close your eyes and concentrate solely on your breathing.

4. Pay attention to your breath as it enters via your nose, exits through your mouth, and enters your diaphragm. Keep your attention on your breathing.

5. As you concentrate on your breathing, various thoughts and feelings will arise. As an alcoholic, you can say to yourself, "I can't believe I'm so addicted to alcohol." Observe these thoughts when they arise. Do not engage in combat with them. Don't cling to them. Simply keep an eye on them. You can also have feelings like a desire for a drink or a glass of wine. Simply examine these ideas and feelings before returning your attention to your breathing.

6. Now I'd like you to start reciting a mantra. "I forgive myself for having an addiction," the slogan goes. Now that I am here, I give myself love, strength, and the ability to heal."

7. Maintain your focus on your breath while chanting this mantra. You will continue to have ideas and feelings, which is perfectly normal. Allow them to come and go as they will, while focusing on your breathing.

8. Keep going for another 20 minutes.

9. Finally, wish yourself, "May I live a happy and healthy life."

This easy activity can help you become more conscious and promote self-forgiveness and compassion. It is the most effective meditation for quitting drinking alcohol.

There are a variety of workouts that can help you quit alcohol. Let's take a closer look.

What should you say to someone who has an alcohol disorder?

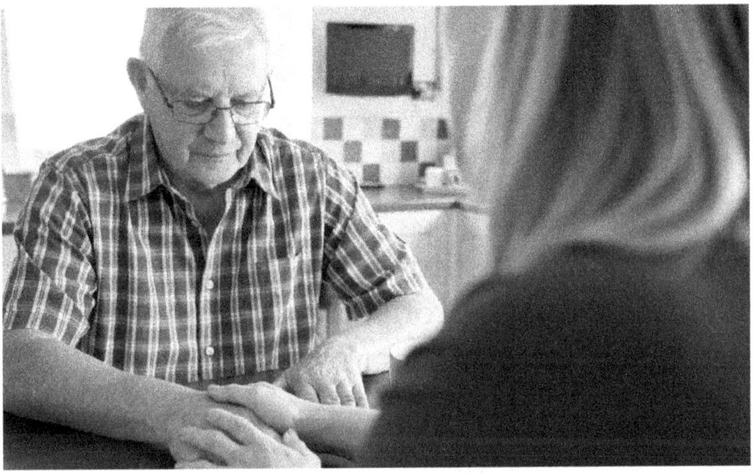

The first step is to educate yourself about alcoholism.

Before you do anything, make sure you know if your friend or loved one is addicted to alcohol. Alcoholism, often known as alcohol use disorder, is more than just drinking too much occasionally. Alcohol as a coping technique or a social habit can appear to be the same as alcoholism, but it is different. Even if they say they're only having one drink, people with alcohol use disorders don't drink responsibly. Read more about the signs and symptoms of alcoholism.

Additional resources and information on supporting someone with an alcohol addiction can be found on government and programme websites. To learn more about the addiction and the experience, take a look at the following resources:

• Al-Anon

• A.A.

• SAMHSA

• The National Institute on Alcohol Abuse and Alcoholism is a non-profit organisation dedicated to preventing and treating alcohol abuse and addiction

Step 2: Rehearse your speech.

Make it known to the individual you care about that you are available and concerned. Make uplifting, encouraging words. Avoid being pessimistic, insensitive, or arrogant.

The use of "I" words reduces accusation and allows you to participate actively in the conversation. Bringing up a specific issue could be beneficial. You might mention a time when alcohol resulted in an unfavourable outcome, such as violent conduct or financial difficulties. Instead of saying, "You're an alcoholic," you may respond, "I love you and you're very essential to me." I'm concerned about the amount of alcohol you're drinking; it could be harmful to your health."

Make sure you're ready for everything. Stay cool and convince your person that you respect and support them, regardless of their attitude.

Step 3: Determine the best time and location for your event.

Pick an appropriate time to hold this crucial discussion. Have the discussion in a location where you can be certain of solitude and silence. You'll also want to avoid any distractions so that you can both focus on each other. Check to see whether your loved one is irritated or concerned with something else. The person should be sober first and foremost.

Step 4: Be honest and compassionate while approaching and listening to others.

If you suspect that the individual has an alcohol issue, the best thing you can do is be open and honest with them about it. It won't help the problem if you hope the person will improve on their own.

Tell your loved one you're concerned they're drinking too much and that you're willing to help. Be ready for a backlash. Make an effort to roll with any pushback to your ideas. It's possible that the person is in denial and will react furiously to your efforts. Take it in stride. Allow them time and space to consider their options before making a decision, and pay attention to what they have to say.

Step 5: Lend a helping hand.

You can't make someone go to treatment if they don't want to. You can only help by offering your assistance. It is up to them to decide whether or not they will accept the offer. Be honest, compassionate, and nonjudgmental. Consider how you would react if you found yourself in the same circumstances.

Your friend or loved one might also make a personal commitment to reduce their consumption. Words aren't as essential as actions, though. Encourage the individual to seek treatment in a formal setting. Inquire about specific promises, and then follow up.

Check with other family members and friends to see if they wish to participate. This depends on a variety of factors, including the gravity of the event and the individual's desire for privacy.

Intervene (Step 6)

An intervention is distinct from approaching someone to discuss your problems. An intervention entails a higher level of commitment. Planning, imposing penalties, sharing, and proposing a treatment choice are all part of the process.

If the person is really resistive to receiving assistance, an intervention may be necessary. Friends, family members, and coworkers gather to confront the person and push them to seek therapy throughout this procedure. Interventions are frequently carried out with the assistance of a qualified counsellor. A qualified therapist can help you with the following:

- offer suggestions on how to get the individual into treatment
- Describe the various treatment choices
- look for local programmes

Treatment is provided free of charge by several authorities and groups.

What Causes People to Relapse?

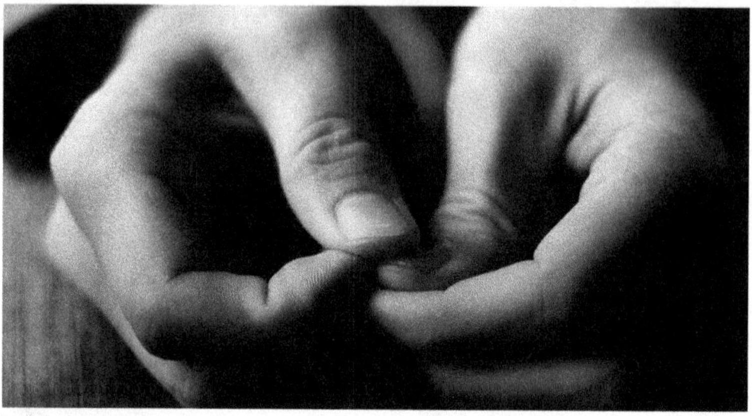

Maintaining your health and sobriety demands a tremendous amount of time and effort. Surprisingly, some people relapse after completing alcohol therapy. Triggers such as a gathering of alcoholic friends, particular exercises, or certain circumstances can cause someone to revert to old drinking habits.
Relapsing doesn't mean you've failed or that you'll never be able to beat alcoholism. It makes you more aware of triggers and may prompt you to seek additional help from a guide or support group. Participating in ongoing treatment tactics gives you a better chance of long-term abstinence than those who do not pursue recovery through maintenance programmes.

Some people relapse for a variety of reasons, including:

- Getting rid of old behaviours

- Anxiety and stress
- Social compulsions
- Instability of mind or emotions
- Anger or irritability
- The want to get intoxicated once more

Treatment is the first step toward a brighter future. Experts in alcohol therapy collaborate with you to create a personalised, long-term recovery plan with measurable goals. Inpatient or outpatient treatment, prescription-assisted treatment, directing, and upkeep gatherings are all possible components of comprehensive recovery plans.

When it comes to alcohol, how long does it stay in your system?

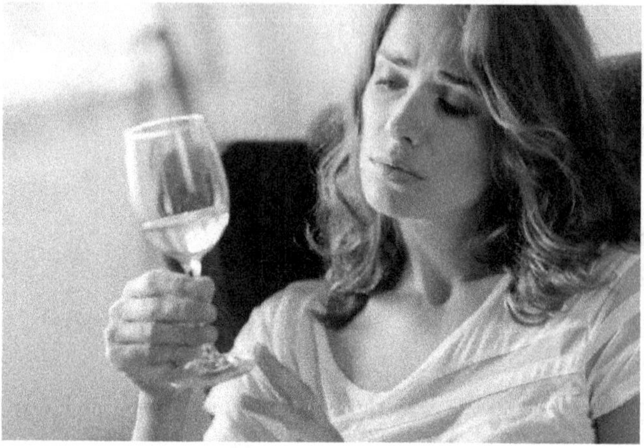

Overview

Alcohol is a depressant with a short half-life in the human body. Your body will begin to metabolise alcohol at a rate of 20 milligrammes per deciliter (mg/dL) per hour once it has entered your system. That indicates that metabolising the alcohol would take roughly two hours if your blood alcohol level was 40 mg/dL.

When the affects of alcohol wear off, how long does it take?

Although alcohol is metabolised at a consistent rate, certain persons may experience its effects for longer periods of time. Because blood alcohol concentrations differ between people and situations, this is the case.

The amount of alcohol in your blood in relation to the amount of water in your blood is referred to as blood alcohol concentration (BAC). If two people have blood alcohol levels of 20 mg/dL, the alcohol will metabolise in each person in about an hour, but their BACs will be considerably different.

BAC and how you react to alcohol are affected by a variety of factors, including:

- age
- weight
- consuming alcoholic beverages on an empty stomach
- medications
- liver ailment
- binge drinking (drinking a large number of drinks in a short period of time)

It's also crucial to know how much alcohol is in your drink, as this will impact how long it takes for your drink to be metabolised. Some beers, for example, have a larger alcohol content, which influences how much alcohol you get from a single drink.

What is the process of metabolising alcohol?

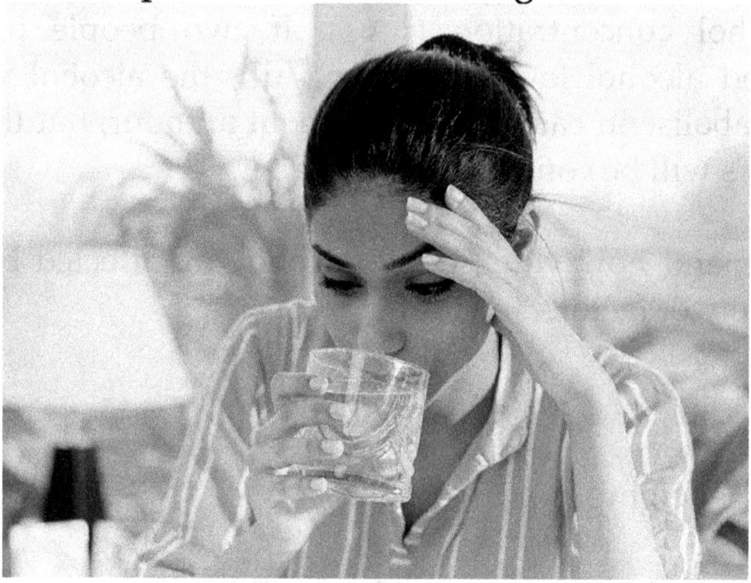

When you drink alcohol, it initially passes through your digestive system. Alcohol, on the other hand, is not metabolised in the same way that food and other beverages are. A single drink delivers about 20% of the alcohol directly to the blood vessels. It then makes its way to your brain. The remaining 80% passes via your small intestine and into your bloodstream.

The liver is responsible for removing alcohol from the body towards the end of its life cycle. This procedure can be slowed down if you have a liver problem.

Tests of urine vs. tests of breath

Urine tests can identify alcohol even if you haven't had a drink in a long time. These tests seek for alcohol metabolite traces. Between 12 and 48 hours after drinking, an average urine test can identify alcohol. Advanced testing can detect alcohol in your urine up to 80 hours after you've consumed alcohol.

Tests for alcohol in the breath Can detect alcohol in a shorter amount of time On average, this takes roughly 24 hours. A breathalyser is a tiny equipment that measures your blood alcohol content (BAC). Any figure greater than 0.02 is deemed dangerous when driving or performing other safety-related tasks.

Alcohol can last up to 90 days in your hair. It can also be identified in saliva, perspiration, and blood for a short period of time.

Alcohol and breastfeeding

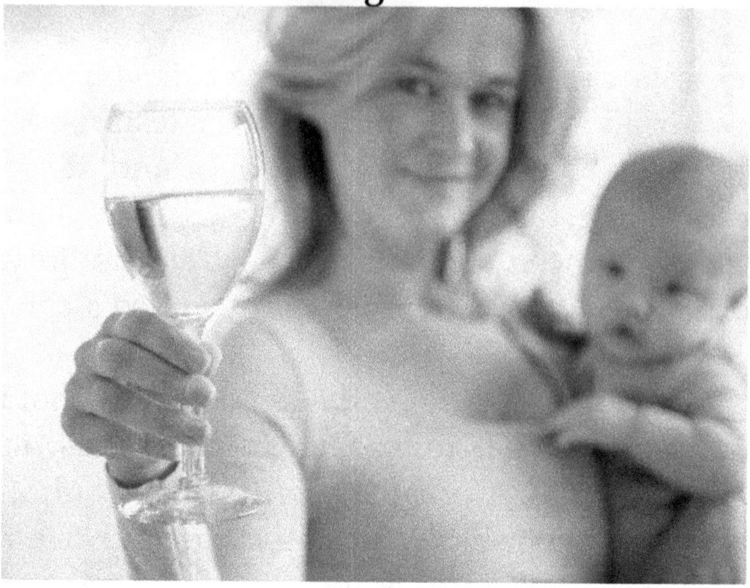

It's a common misperception that keeping track of how much alcohol you drink and how long it takes your body to get rid of it might help keep breast milk healthy. When you're breastfeeding, no quantity of alcohol is safe to drink. Babies who have been exposed to alcohol are more likely to have delayed motor skills and other developmental issues.

While the Mayo Clinic claims that alcohol clears breast milk in a few hours on average, the process varies just like it does for women who aren't breastfeeding.

If you do decide to drink alcohol while breastfeeding, keep the following tips in mind:

- Don't drink anything until you've breastfed.

• Prepare extra milk ahead of time so you may feed your baby expressed milk.

• After a shot or a 12-ounce drink of alcohol or wine, wait 2-3 hours before breastfeeding again.

Poisoning by alcohol

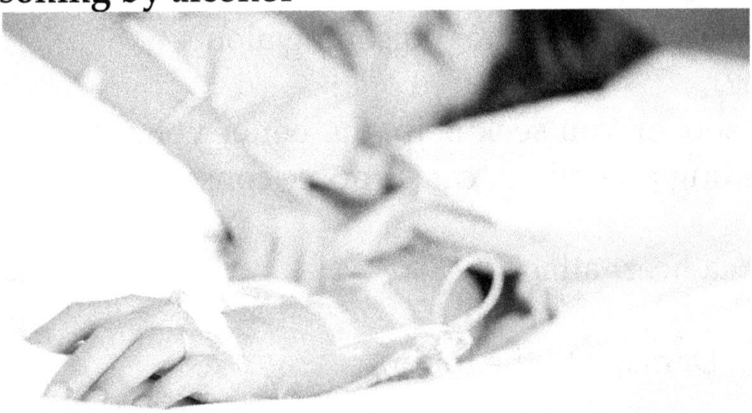

Alcohol poisoning is a serious medical disease that requires immediate medical attention. It happens when you drink a lot of alcohol and your body can't break it down fast enough. The most common cause of alcohol toxicity is binge drinking.

Among the signs and symptoms are:

- vomiting
- lowered body temperature
- Breathing more slowly

- being thrown out

Alcohol poisoning often causes a person to pass out before they realise what has happened. If you suspect a friend or loved one is suffering from alcohol poisoning, contact your local emergency services right once. Turn the person on their side to avoid choking on vomit. Never leave a buddy who is suffering from alcohol poisoning alone.

The sooner you seek help, the better your chances of avoiding potentially catastrophic consequences like:

- a heart attack
- Damage to the brain
- seizure
- asphyxiation
- blood pressure that is dangerously low

How long do you think it'll take you to feel better?

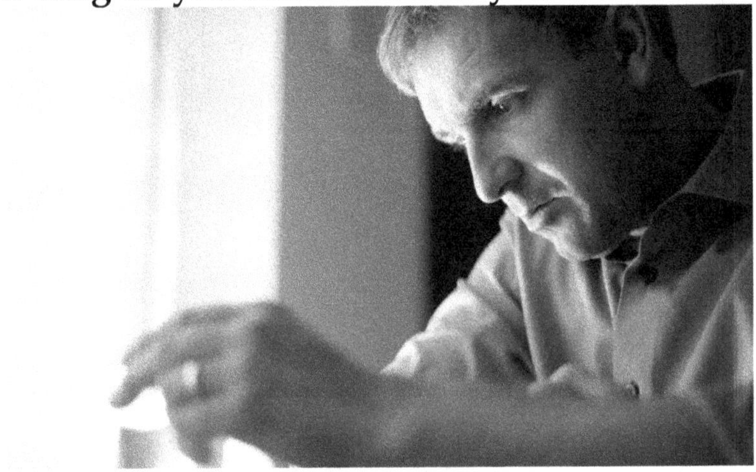

Each and every one of us is unique. Withdrawal from alcohol is different for everyone; there is no such thing as "normal," and it might be difficult to predict an individual's experience. No doctor will be able to say how long it will take for the advantages to become apparent. Some people report great results in as little as a week, while others claim it took over six months for them to feel like themselves again. Emotions, sleep, and overall health patterns all require time to adjust, and this is typically tied to the amount of alcohol consumed, your general health prior to quitting drinking, and even environmental and emotional factors that might influence the process of quitting drinking.

Although not everyone who stops drinking alcohol gets the same withdrawal symptoms, many people who have been drinking for a long time, often, or heavily will experience withdrawal if they stop abruptly. The following are the most common signs and symptoms:

Psychological Signs and Symptoms

- Anxiety
- Nightmares
- Depression
- Inability to think clearly
- Fatigue
- Are you jittery or nervous?
- Irritability or a proclivity for ecstasy
- Emotional shifts that happen quickly
- Shakiness

Physical Signs and Symptoms

- Hypertension (high blood pressure)
- Insomnia
- Headaches

- Appetite loss.

- Palpitations or a fast heart rate

- Sweating, particularly on the palms of your hands or on the face

- Tremors

Changes in sleep habits, tiredness, and mood swings, for example, can linger for weeks or even months. However, five to seven days after you quit drinking, you should start to feel better.

Why do we feel worse before we feel better when we quit smoking?

Alcohol slows your brain since it is a depressant. When a person drinks often, frequently, or for an extended period of time, the brain compensates by generating more stimulating chemicals to counteract the depressing effects (compared to when a person does not drink). The brain's new normal is overproduction.

When someone quits drinking, their brain continues to produce additional chemicals, which can lead to the unpleasant alcohol withdrawal symptoms associated with overstimulation. The mind will adjust, but a person in withdrawal may feel poorly until it does. This frequently leads to a recurrence, so understanding why you're sick and that the symptoms are only temporary is critical to getting through it.

Depression

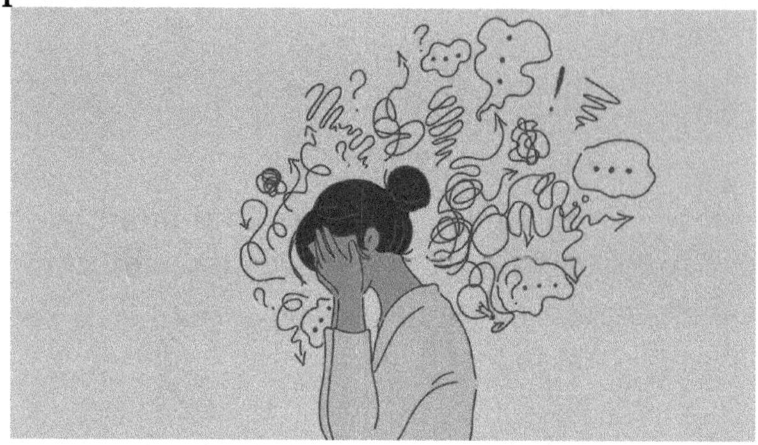

Depression and alcohol are linked in a variety of ways. Some people develop alcoholism as a result of depression, whereas others develop it as a result of drinking. Some people experience depression after quitting alcohol. So, what's the point of becoming sober if you're only going to feel worse? However, most cases of post-alcoholic sadness are very transient. Alcohol withdrawal, for example, might result in depressive symptoms. Furthermore, you may require some time to acclimatise to life without alcohol.

Although it does not affect everyone, depression is a common side effect of abstaining from alcohol. After quitting alcohol, even moderate drinkers experience depression. It can occur for a variety of reasons, but if left unattended, it can lead to relapse.

When you stop drinking, your body undergoes chemical changes. Alcohol affects a variety of physiological systems and nearly every neurotransmitter. After you stop numbing your brain with alcohol, it practically goes into hyperdrive for a moment. Realistically, it could take anything from a few months to a year to reestablish a baseline and feel better.

Emotional Healing

There is a psychological adjustment period once you stop drinking. You've let go of your shield and now need to deal with those difficulties and anxieties before moving forward. When answering the question, "How long does it take to feel better after you quit drinking?" this can be a wild card.

All of the reasons you drank remain. With the alcohol, you simply numbed them. Now you must determine the source of your anxiety and despair, as well as how you will cope without the use of alcohol. When you use alcohol to dull your emotions and then stop, you're forced to confront a lot of truths about your life that you've been ignoring for years. That's terrifying, and it's also emotionally draining.

You may have used alcohol as a coping method when things got difficult when you were drinking. That isn't the case now. As a result, when issues arise, you may find yourself unable to cope as effectively as before. When you quit alcohol, the increased stress, combined with any other events, might lead to some perplexing situations.

Try to remember yourself that every challenge you confront and overcome without the use of alcohol will build your confidence; nevertheless, you must do it in order to receive the good feedback. As a result, take on the easier difficulties first, then go on to the more difficult ones later.

Alcoholism Addiction Treatment with Natural Remedies

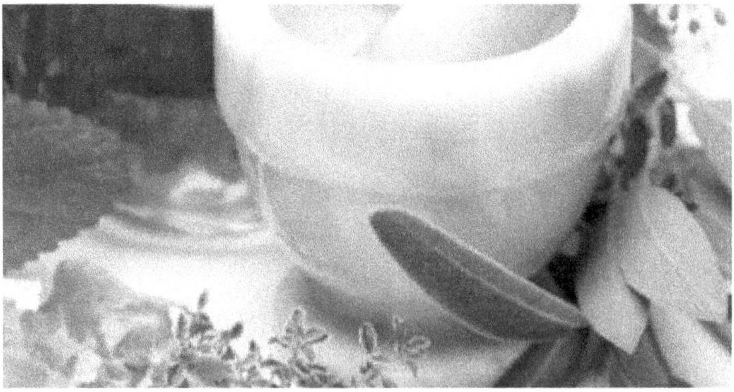

Alcoholism is a term that is widely used to describe an alcohol consumption disorder (AUD). Treatment and recovery from this addiction are challenging processes that require a lot of consistent support.

While it's not a good idea to rely primarily on alternative therapies or remedies for this, some natural approaches, including as meditation, acupuncture, and some medicines, may help you feel better as you progress through these stages.

If you're thinking about using any of the following approaches, make sure to talk to your doctor about the potential benefits and hazards.

- **Acupuncture**

Acupuncture is a needle-based therapy that has been utilised in traditional Chinese medicine for thousands of years (TCM). It's usually advised for reducing alcohol cravings, alleviating withdrawal symptoms, and easing the anxiety and despair that come with alcoholism. Acupuncture is now being studied to see if it is beneficial for this aim.

A meta-analysis of research indicated that acupuncture treatment had a stronger effect on lowering alcohol cravings and withdrawal, as well as alcohol-related behaviours, than sham acupuncture (needles placed into non-specific areas instead of those considered to target alcohol use disorder).

This was determined on the final post-treatment checkup. In the long run, however, the effect was minimal. The National Acupuncture Detoxification Program (NADA), which incorporates ear acupuncture, is a treatment strategy for addiction.

- **Extract of Kudzu**

Kudzu extract has shown some potential in lowering consumption and moderating binge drinking in heavy drinkers who are not seeking treatment for alcoholism. The main ingredient in the TCM formula ge hai jie cheng tang is kudzu flower (ge hua), which has long been used to treat alcohol intoxication (and hangover).

It has a number of impacts, including increasing blood alcohol levels more quickly, making you feel inebriated sooner. It is also thought to prevent the clearance of acetaldehyde, an alcohol breakdown product with undesirable side effects. Antabuse (disulfiram), a medication licenced for the treatment of alcoholism, provides the similar advantage.

For a 90-minute session of drinking beer, binge drinkers were given either kudzu extract or a placebo.

The patients who were given a single dosage of kudzu extract drank considerably less beer than those who were given a placebo or their baseline measurement. They also drank more slowly.

In a study of heavy drinkers who refused to enter a treatment programme, kudzu extract had no effect on their alcohol cravings. It did, however, lower the number of drinks they consumed each week by a third to half, reduce the number of heavy drinking days, and raise the proportion and number of abstinent days.

- **Ashwagandha**

Ashwagandha is a herbal supplement derived from the Withania somnifera plant that has been used in

Ayurvedic therapy for alcohol withdrawal and cravings for centuries. Trials on alcohol-addicted rodents have shown that it can help with anxiety, but more human studies are needed to corroborate this.

- **Thistle (Milk)**

Milk thistle (Silybum marianum), a herb high in the antioxidant silymarin, is frequently promoted as a way to improve liver function and prevent alcohol-induced liver damage.

While preliminary study suggests that milk thistle may be useful in the treatment of alcohol-related liver damage, additional research is needed before definitive conclusions can be drawn about the herb's efficacy in improving liver health.

• **Drinking a Lot of Water to Break the Alcohol Habit**

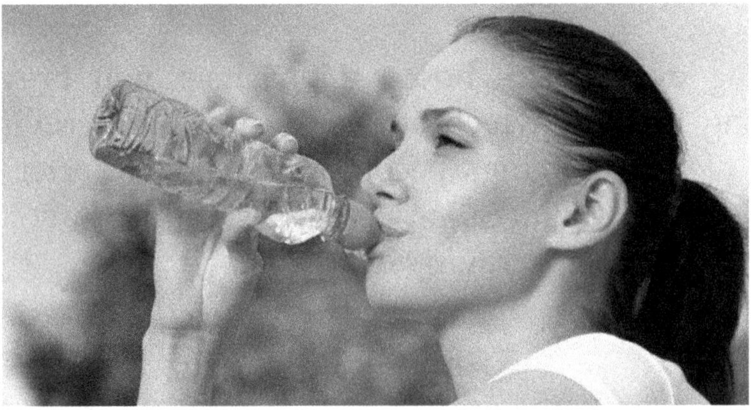

We are all aware that water is beneficial to our health and that we should drink eight glasses every day. If you're looking for natural ways to stop drinking alcohol, you've discovered the most effective method: drink plenty of water.

When you quit alcohol, your body becomes dehydrated, and you feel nauseated. By draining toxins out of your body, drinking water not only hydrates you but also reduces the tremors and alcohol cravings. While electrolyte-rich sports drinks can be added, never drink more than 2 quarts of fluid per hour.

• **Alcohol Cravings are reduced by Eating a Healthy Diet**

Eating a balanced diet is a great natural strategy to stop alcohol cravings. Lean proteins like chicken, eggs, and fish are part of a healthy diet. Fresh fruits and vegetables, potatoes, legumes, and whole grains are all included.

Eating every three hours might help you prevent feeling hungry, which can lead to alcohol cravings. The alcohol cravings become more severe after the tremors take hold. Sugary snacks should be avoided to reduce alcohol cravings.

- **Remedy with whole grains, nuts, dates, and seeds**

You'll want to eat nutritious grains like barley, brown rice, almonds, cashews, or Brazilian nuts to keep your blood sugar stable. Controlling your alcohol cravings might be as simple as eating sunflower seeds or a banana. Dates are a dependable supply of sugar that will quench your thirst. Crushing some dates and combining them with water has been shown to help lessen alcohol cravings. Drink this blend at least twice a day or whenever you're drinking something sweet.

- **Remedies combining herbs and liquids**

Three parts thyme roots, two parts knotgrass tops, and one part wormwood tops added to boiling water is another natural cure I discovered. It's possible that drinking this will aid with alcohol withdrawal. Kudzu, golden root, and passion flower are among natural herbs that have been reported to aid in the cessation of drinking. These herbs can help you overcome your alcohol addiction and lessen your use.

- **Primrose of the Evening**

By controlling your digestion, evening primrose aids in the reduction of alcohol cravings. Our intestines are infested with bacteria. Long-term alcohol consumption causes the bacteria in the digestive tract to accumulate toxins, which causes you to crave alcohol. Evening primrose can help drain that bacteria out of your system, reducing cravings and allowing you to stop smoking more quickly. It's available as an oil. Take three drops three times a day for three weeks, either straight or mixed with water.

History of smoking

The first use of smoking in shamanism dates back to 5000 BC in the Americas. European arrivals in the 16th century brought rapid expansion of tobacco cultivation, use, and trade. With the rebuilding of agriculture and industry, cigarettes became more easily available in the U.S. following the rebuilding period. Mass production rapidly broadened the reach of consumption, which increased until the 1960s scientific debates and criticism.

Cannabis and other plants were formerly evaporated on hot rocks or charcoal, burnt as incense or in containers and censers, and breathed indirectly. Direct smoking before to the 16th century is debatable, with pipes believed to have been used to smoke cannabis dating from the 10th to 12th centuries discovered in Southeastern Africa.

Previously used for medical purposes, cocaine smoking became popular in China and the West throughout the nineteenth century. These events resulted in the development of opium dens. Opium smoking became widespread in Europe's creative circles in the later part of the century. While gambling dens persisted across the globe, the tendency among Europeans slowed throughout World War I, and even among Chinese during the Cultural Revolution.

During the 1920s, increasing cigarette use and life span made the negative health consequences more apparent. Fritz Lickint of Dresden, Germany, presented solid statistical proof of a lung cancer–tobacco connection in 1929, sparking a major anti-smoking campaign in Nazi Germany. The topic remained virtually taboo until 1954, when the British Doctors Study was published, and until 1964, when the United States Surgeon General issued a report. Smoking became stigmatized, resulting in the Tobacco Master Settlement Agreement (MSA), the biggest civil settlement in US history, in

1998.

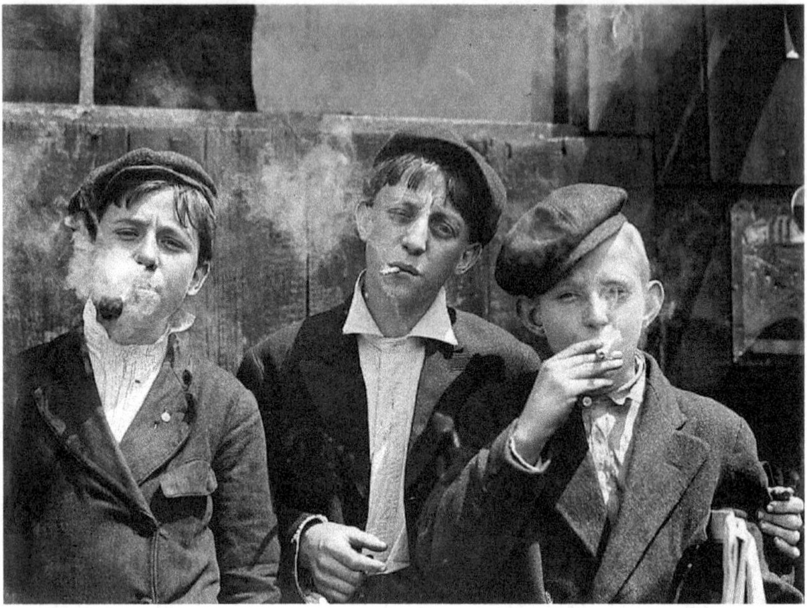

Usage in ancient times

Since ancient times, people have smoked in some form or another. Tobacco and other hallucinogenic substances were smoked in shamanistic ceremonies across the Americas as early as 5000 BC, and they originated in the Peruvian and Ecuadorian Andes. Incense was used in religious ceremonies by many ancient civilizations, including the Babylonians, Indians, and Chinese, as well as the Israelites and subsequent Catholic and Orthodox churches. However, burning incense does not result in direct inhalation. It has been claimed that cannabis resin, or perhaps opium, was used in this incense at times [citation required]. It is unclear how much cannabis resin was in this incense and if it originated from psychotropic cannabis or perhaps opium. Cannabis vapours were used by the ancient Assyrians to treat "poison of the limbs," which was assumed to be arthritis.

According to the Greek historian Herodotus', the Scythians smoked cannabis seeds as part of their cultural rites. He wrote this after seeing a burial procession for one of their kings:

They construct a booth by laying three sticks inclined towards one another on the ground and wrapping woolen felts around them, arranging them so that they fit as closely as possible: inside the booth, a dish is placed on the ground into which a number of red-hot stones are placed, followed by hemp seed. It immediately starts to smoke, emitting a vapour unrivalled by any vapor-bath in Greece. The Scythians rejoiced and shouted for joy.

Scythians built sweat lodges, which many peoples utilized for ritual purposes. There was a smaller replica of a Scythian burial site discovered in the Tien Shen Mountains by Sergei Ivanovich Rudenko in 1947-1949. Tent poles were encased in a leather bag that contained cannabis seed. There are also coriander seeds in this Kurgan. The smoke for ceremonial bathing was most likely created by evaporating cannabis seeds and coriander seeds on hot rocks.

For social or religious reasons (which varied between cultures), pipe smoking was the most common type of smoking among indigenous peoples in early North America. Representatives of rival tribes would smoke pipes, and later European settlers would smoke them, as a gesture of good will, diplomacy, or peace (thus the nickname, "peace pipe"). As early as the Caribbean, Mexico, Central and South America, smoking reeds or cigars was the most common smoking equipment.

In recent years, pipes have become increasingly popular. As early as the 9th century, smoking is visible in engravings and on different kinds of ceramics, though it isn't known whether smoking was restricted to the upper class or only the priestly class.

As Europeans arrived in America during the late 15th century, tobacco smoking became popular as a leisure activity. An Aztec feast would begin with the serving of fragrant flowers and smoking tubes to the dining guests. At the conclusion of the banquet, which lasted all night, any leftover flowers, smoking tubes, and food would be distributed as charity to the elderly and needy attendees. They would also be awarded to the servers.

Smoking prevalence

Europe

Dirck Hals, 1627, Gentlemen Smoking and Playing Backgammon in an Interior. Tobacco was brought to France from Spain in 1560 by a Frenchman called Jean Nicot (from whence the term nicotine originates). It spread from there to England. The first reported smoking Englishman was a seaman in Bristol in 1556, who was observed "emitting smoke from his nose." Tobacco, like tea, coffee, and opium, was one of several intoxicants that were initially employed as a kind of medicine.

Early modern European medical research was still heavily founded on humorism, the belief that everything had a distinct humoral character that differed between hot and cold, dry and wet. Tobacco was often seen as helpful because to its heating and drying qualities, and an infinite number of positive attributes was ascribed to it. The idea of consuming chemicals in the form of smoke was likewise novel, and Europeans reacted with surprise and mistrust.

The argument raged among priests, scientists, and laypeople over whether tobacco was a curse or a blessing, and both sides had strong advocates. The English monarch, James I, was one of the earliest vocal doubters, publishing A Counterblast to Tobacco, an unforgiving literary attack on what he saw as a societal threat. Though replete with, at times, irrelevant and incomplete arguments, it did address some of the health concerns and highlighted the odd reality that tobacco was often given contradictory, and at times seemingly miraculous, properties:

It sobers up a guy who was previously inebriated. It restores a tired guy while also making him hungry. When eaten before going to bed, it induces deep slumber; but, when taken when a man is sleepy and drowsy, it will, as they say, awaken his brain and accelerate his intellect. It is used to cure the Pocks, but only among the pocked Indian slaves. It is polished in England, and will not deign to treat anything except cleanly and gentlemanly illnesses.

Southeast Asia and South Asia

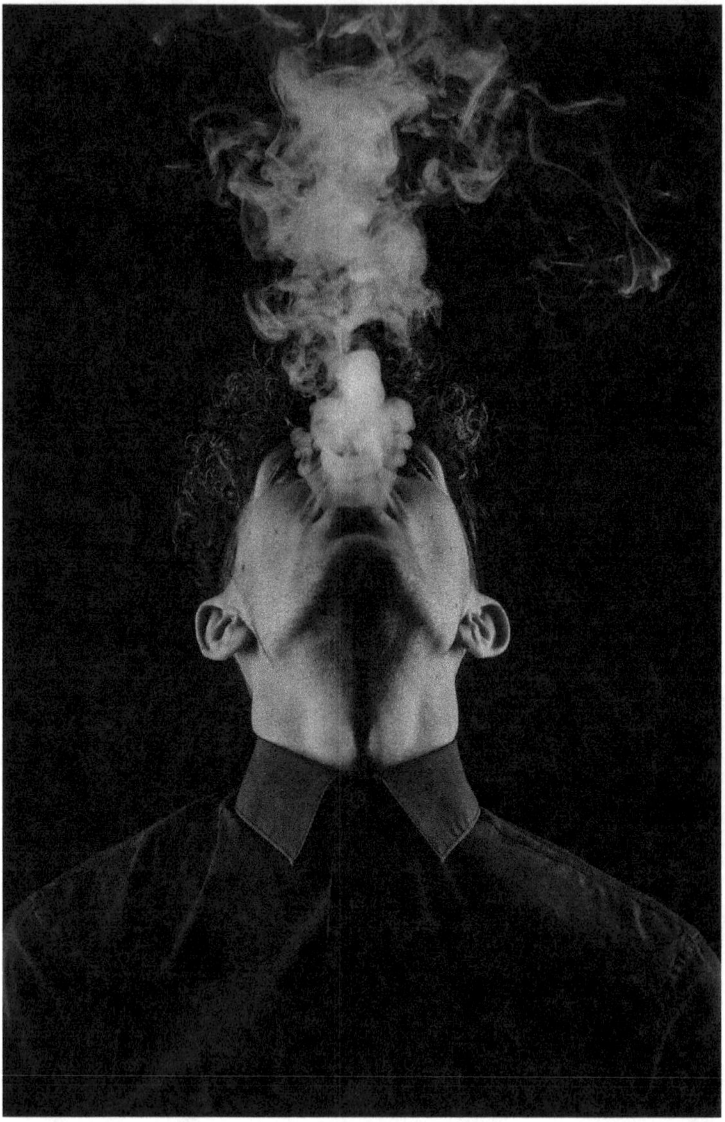

Cannabis 'smoking' in India has been known from at least 2000 BC and is first referenced in the

Atharvaveda, which dates back a few hundred years BC. Fumigation (dhupa) and fire offerings (homa) are medically recommended in Ayurveda and have been performed for at least 3,000 years, while smoking, dhumrapana (literally "drinking smoke"), has been practiced for at least 2,000 years. Rather of being smoked in a pipe or wrapped into a cigarette, the cannabis was always burnt in an open vessel or censer.

Fumigation and fire offerings have been carried out using a variety of materials, including clarified butter (ghee), fish offal, dried snake skins, and different pastes molded around incense sticks and burned to disperse smoke over large distances. Inhaling smoke was used as a treatment for a wide range of illnesses. It was not restricted to cannabis, but included other plants and medical mixtures suggested to improve general health.

Prior to the contemporary era, smoking was done using pipes with varying lengths of stems, known as chillums. Dhumrapana has been almost completely supplanted by cigarette smoking nowadays, although dhupa and homa are still performed. A contemporary descendent of the ancient dhumrapana is beady, a kind of hand rolled herbal cigarette made of cloves, powdered betel nut, and tobacco, typically in a low percentage of tobacco.

In the early 1880s, kretek, a kind of cigarette containing cloves, was developed in Indonesia as a means of delivering the medicinal benefits of clove oil, or eugenol, to the lungs. It soon became a popular cough medicine, and in the early twentieth century, kretek, manufacturers started selling pre-rolled clove cigarettes. Kretek became a national emblem in the 1960s and 1970s, with tax advantages compared to "white" cigarettes, and manufacturing started to move from traditional hand-rolling to machine-rolling.

In the mid-1980s, the industrial technique surpassed the hand-rolled method in terms of volume, and now, kretek controls up to 90% of the Indonesian cigarette market. The manufacturing is one of the biggest sources of revenue for the Indonesian government, and the production, which is distributed among 500 independent producers, directly employs 180,000 people and indirectly employs over 10 million.

The Arab World

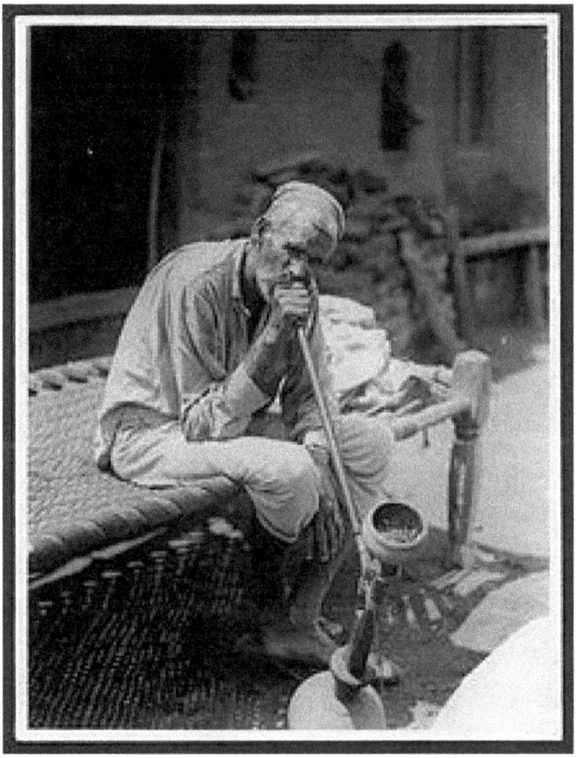

Muhammad Qasim's painting of a Persian girl smoking. Isfahan in the 17th century.

Water pipes were brought into Persia and the Middle East from China in the 16th century. Initially, these pipes were used to smoke tobacco, but cannabis flowers and hashish were soon added. As tobacco usage expanded in the Middle East and Northern Africa, the hashish trade exploded in a matter of decades. Hashish smoking rapidly gained popularity throughout Eurasia, from Turkey to Nepal, during the 16th and 17th centuries, culminating in the late 19th and early 20th centuries. Throughout the 18th century, the method of collecting and drying cannabis plants to produce hashish grew more common as mass manufacturing became essential to meet the rapidly expanding Eurasian hashish trade.

As they do today, pipes frequently featured several tubes to accommodate multiple smokers, or users would pass the nozzle around in the many smoking establishments that served as social centers in major Muslim cultural centers such as Istanbul, Baghdad, and Cairo. Smoking, particularly with the introduction of tobacco, became an integral component of Muslim society and culture, being interwoven with major rituals like as weddings and funerals and manifesting itself in architecture, dress, literature, and poetry.

There is a mention to tobacco in a Persian poetry dated before 1536, but the validity of the text has been called into doubt due to a lack of supporting references. The next credible eyewitness account of tobacco smoking comes from a Spanish ambassador in 1617, but by then the habit had been firmly ingrained in Persian culture.

Persia was the birthplace of the Argila (or hookah). The rich's pipes were constructed of beautifully crafted glass and precious metals, while the poor folk utilized coconuts with bamboo tubing to smoke cannabis before the introduction of tobacco.

The mixture of the two drugs became extremely popular, and it was even smoked in regular "dry" pipes. The water-pipe, on the other hand, remained the most popular smoking instrument until the invention of the cigarette in the twentieth century. Foreign visitors to the area often commented on how prevalent smoking was among Persians. During Ramadan, the Muslim fasting season during which no food is consumed while the sun is up, one of the first things many Persians performed after nightfall was fire their pipes.

Both sexes smoked, but for women smoking was a private pleasure enjoyed in the privacy of their own houses. Iran was one of the world's biggest tobacco exporters in the nineteenth century, and the habit had already established a national Iranian characteristic.

The East Asian region

Tobacco came to Asia when Europeans discovered the Americas, first through Spanish and Portuguese sailors, then by the Dutch and English. Spain and Portugal were active in Central and South America, where cigarettes and cigars were the preferred smoking equipment, and its sailors mainly smoked cigars. The English and Dutch became acquainted with the pipe-smoking inhabitants of North America and adopted the practice. While Southern Europeans started smoking earlier, it was the northerners' long-stemmed pipes that became popular throughout East and Southeast Asia. Tobacco smoking was introduced in the Philippines by expatriates as early as the 1570s.

By the early 17th century, the kiseru, a long-stemmed Japanese pipe influenced by Dutch clay pipes, had become popular enough to be included in Buddhist children's text books. Tobacco smoking developed as a component of the Japanese tea ceremony by repurposing several of the traditional incense-burning objects for tobacco smoking. The k-bon (incense tray) developed into the tobacco-bon, the incense burner became a pot for tobacco embers, and the incense pot into an ash tray.

Weapons were widely employed as items of ostentation throughout the Edo era, signifying wealth and social position. Because only samurai were permitted to carry weapons, an ornate kiseru hung about the waist performed a similar function. Following the Meiji restoration and the abolition of the caste system, many artisans who had previously adorned swords moved to creating kiserus and tobacco bag buckles. Though mass-production of cigarettes started in the late 1800s, it wasn't until after World War II that the kiseru fell out of favor, becoming a symbol of tradition and relative obscurity.

Social stigmatization

Historic dissent

Since smoking was introduced outside of the Americas, it has been met with fierce resistance. Arguments varied from socioeconomic—tobacco was referred to as a usurper of excellent agricultural land—to simply moralistic, with many religiously devoted people seeing tobacco as another kind of sinful drunkenness. Many reasons were given to the effect that smoking was dangerous, and even though the critics were ultimately correct in many of their assertions, the objections were seldom founded on scientific reasoning, and if they were, they often depended on humorist and other pre-modern scientific techniques.

Tobacco, according to Dr. Eleazar Duncon, "...is so harmful and hazardous to youth that it may have the poisonous nation stated in the name, and that it were as well known by the name of Youths-bane as by the name of tobacco."

Tobacconists and smokers are portrayed in early 17th century descriptive notes of different distinctive kinds and styles of men as people who suffer from erroneous self-images and misguided beliefs about the characteristics of tobacco use.

Though doctors such as Benjamin Rush stated that tobacco use (including smoking) was harmful to health as early as 1798, it wasn't until the early twentieth century that researchers began to undertake significant medical investigations.

Politics undergoing a renaissance

The invention of mechanized tobacco equipment occurred in the late nineteenth century. Factories, mainly in the southern United States, enabled low-cost mass manufacturing of cigarettes. As the Victorian period gave way to the Edwardian, cigarettes became more elegant and popular among society men. Dr. Isaac Adler of the United States was the first to firmly propose that smoking causes lung cancer in 1912.

Prior to World War I, lung cancer was an uncommon illness that few doctors encountered in their careers. Moreover, the significant increase in lung cancer associated with the postwar surge in cigarette smoking prompted early studies into the connection between smoking and cancer. Fritz Lickint of Dresden, Germany, presented a formal statistical explanation of a lung cancer–tobacco connection in 1929, based on a research that found lung cancer patients were more likely to be smokers. Lickint also contended that tobacco usage was the best explanation for why males were four or five times more likely than women to get lung cancer (since women smoked much less).

In Germany, anti-smoking organizations, typically linked with anti-liquor organizations, initially published anti-tobacco use propaganda in the magazine Der Tabakgegner (The Tobacco Opponent), published by the Bohemian organization between 1912 and 1932. The Deutsche Tabakgegner (German Tobacco Opponents) was the second magazine on the topic, published in Dresden from 1919 until 1935.

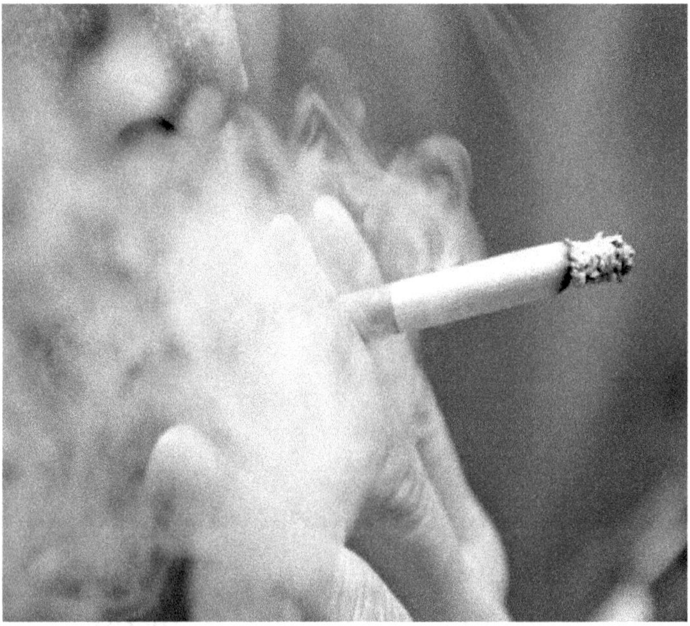

The following compounds are found in cigarette smoke:

The drug nicotine

Tobacco in cigarettes contains nicotine, which is inhaled. Blood flow to the brain is stimulated by the drug. It's easy to become addicted to nicotine.

The symptoms that you typically experience if you are a regular smoker are:

- Appetite.
- Tension.
- Disorientation.
- Lightheadedness.
- Mood swings.
- Crave.
- It's hard to concentrate.
- Drowsiness.
- Nausea.
- A nicotine desire.
- having panic attacks.

The next cigarette alleviates these sensations. This is how nicotine addiction is defined.

The majority of habitual smokers are hooked to nicotine and smoke on a daily basis to feel "normal" and to avoid nicotine withdrawal symptoms.

Addiction initial symptoms within a few hours after the final smoke. Side effects worsen if they are not alleviated by the following smoking. If you stop smoking, the side effects will peak after 3 h and then progressively fade over the next 2-4 weeks.

Approximately two-thirds of smokers desire to quit, yet many fail to do so without assistance. The primary reason why these smokers succeed, despite their desire to quit, is that nicotine addiction is powerful and tough to overcome.

What to do first:

Friends or family often encourage smokers to start. The reason they continue to smoke is nicotine, a chemical found in cigarettes and smokeless tobacco.

In addition to being a stimulant, nicotine is a depressant. The increase in heart rate causes people to become more alert at first. Eventually, it causes fatigue and depression. When people lose their energy and feel depressed and fatigued, as well as when they stop taking nicotine, they need to smoke another cigarette. Nicotine may be as addictive as cocaine and heroin, according to some experts.

It is not impossible to stop smoking permanently; millions of people have already done so. If you want to quit, you can follow these tips:

- **Write it down.**

Writing down your goal improves your chances of success when making a change. If you quit smoking, list all the benefits you'll receive, such as saving money and having more stamina to play sports. Your list should be visible to you. Feel free to add further reasons as they occur to you.

- **You can get help.**

Those who receive support from friends and family have a greater chance of quitting. To help you quit smoking, ask friends if you don't want to disclose that you smoke to your family. Trust an adult you trust and confide in them. Consider joining an online or in-person support group if you have trouble finding people who support you (for example, if your friends smoke and don't want to quit).

Why is it so hard to quit?

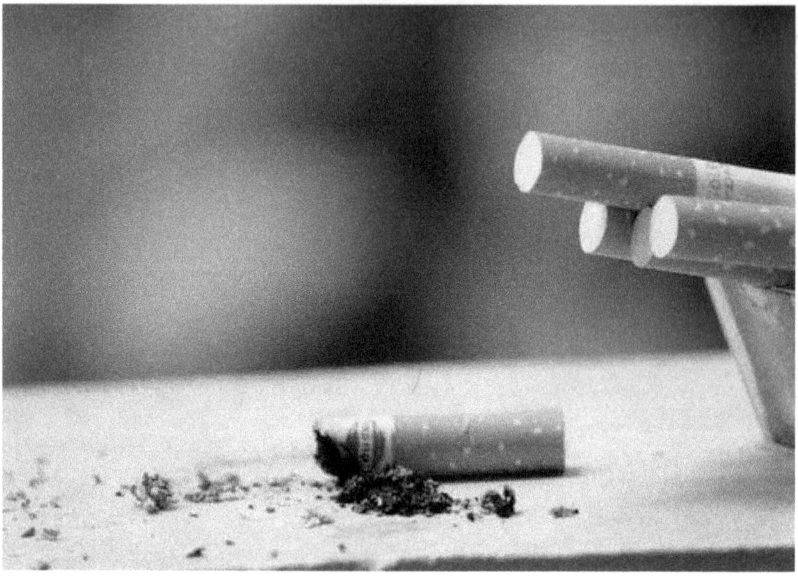

We are all aware of the dangers of smoking, but it doesn't make it any easier to give up the habit altogether. Whether you've been a smoker since you were a youngster or have been a lifelong pack-a-day smoker, quitting may be very difficult.

In addition to being a physical addiction, tobacco use is also a psychological habit. Smoking produces a temporary—and addictive—high due to the nicotine in the cigarettes. When you stop getting your nicotine fix on a regular basis, your body experiences physical withdrawal symptoms and cravings. It is possible that you may resort to cigarettes as a fast and dependable method to improve your perspective, reduce stress, and relax as a result of nicotine's "feel good" impact on the brain. Smoking may also be a coping mechanism for those suffering from despair, anxiety, or simply boredom. Quitting involves discovering new, better methods to deal with the emotions that are causing you distress.

Smoking is also entrenched as a part of one's everyday routine. It's possible that smoking a cigarette with your morning coffee, at a break at work or school, or on your drive home at the end of a long day has become second nature to you. Alternatively, maybe your friends, family, or coworkers smoke, and it has been ingrained in your manner of relating to them.

To effectively quit smoking, you'll need to address both the addiction itself as well as the behaviors and routines that have developed as a result of the addiction. However, it is possible. Anyone who wants to stop smoking may do it with the proper assistance and a well-thought-out plan—even if they've tried and failed many times before.

What is your driving force?

Identifying your why may assist you in staying motivated when times are difficult. People have a variety of reasons for quitting smoking; the following are some of the more frequent ones; however, you may have more. Consider which ones are most effective for you..

Benefits are felt nearly immediately

You will begin to experience the advantages of stopping almost immediately, as your body begins to heal itself. After you stop smoking, you will start seeing results a week to two after you stop.

During the first month

- Carbon monoxide is removed from your bloodstream within 12 hours
- The majority of nicotine has been eliminated from your body in 5 days
- Taste and smell improve within a week

- Within a month, you can expect to see an improvement in your skin

During the first year

- The extra phlegm your lungs produce as a result of smoking will disappear after two months
- The blood flow to your lungs will improve after 3 months
- You have reduced your heart disease risk by half in just 12 months

In the long run, it is more beneficial

- Your stroke risk has dramatically decreased over the past five years
- Your lung cancer risk in 10 years decreases by more than half from that of a continuing smoker--and continues to decline
- Heart attacks and strokes are almost as likely to happen in 15 years as if you had never smoked

○ Health risks can be reduced

You can quit at any time. In order to protect and improve their health, most smokers should stop smoking.

If your body has been damaged, there are some things you can do to reverse it:

- ### Inflammation of the lungs

CilMucus and dirt are removed from the lungs by cilia, which are hairlike projections from certain cells. It is possible to recover from paralysis (but not destruction). Conditions of the chest and lungs exacerbated by smoking, such as asthma and chest infections, can also be improved.

- ### A cancerous condition

Following a total cessation of smoking, the risk of developing most types of cancer is reduced. The earlier you give up smoking, the less chance you have of developing smoking-related cancers.

- ### Irritation of the eyes

It is usually impossible to reverse the damage caused by smoking to the eyes. The damage appears to happen slowly over many years, but it is hard to pinpoint when it occurs.

- ### Your teeth can be damaged

In addition to improving your dental health, quitting smoking will improve your overall health. However, it might take decades for the rate of tooth loss to reach a non-smoker's level after quitting smoking.

The mental health of smokers may be improved by quitting

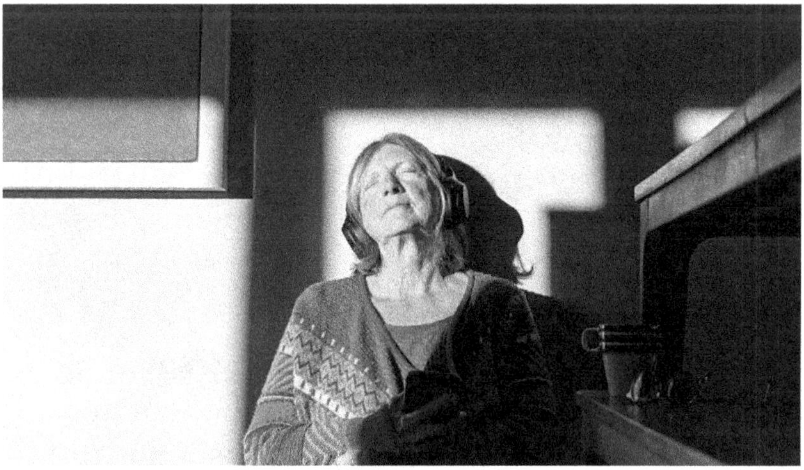

- Several systematic reviews have found that quitting smoking can boost one's health within a matter of weeks.
- Compared to people who did not quit smoking, people who did quit were less likely to experience anxiety, depression, or stress symptoms.

Approximately 480,000 Americans die each year from smoking cigarettes, and 8 million worldwide. Moreover, the World Health Organization (WHO) reports that smoking leads to serious illnesses, poverty, and early death worldwide.

Over the past 50 years, smoking rates have declined substantially, especially in high-income countries, and currently tobacco use is 19.7% in the U.S. Contrary to this, the rate for people with mental health issues remains stubbornly high (36.7%). Mental health practitioners as well as smokers believe smoking reduces stress and anxiety. In the mental health profession, 40–45% of staff believe smoking cessation isn't helpful for patients.

There is also the belief that quitting smoking will worsen mental health symptoms. Smokers are often scared that they will lose relationships after quitting, either because of irritability related to quitting or because they see smoking as a central element of their social life.

Nearly 40 million people continue to smoke cigarettes in the United States, according to the Centers for Disease Control and Prevention (CDC).

Dr. Gemma Taylor, the lead author of the study, explained that many smokers believe cigarettes will help them feel better when they are low. However, there is compelling evidence that smoking actually leads to worse symptoms.

In order to feel good about themselves, it is understandable that people wake up craving cigarettes, satisfy those cravings through smoking, only to want another after hours later.

She continued, "The good news is that better mental health is on the other side of withdrawal." We see a similar link between quitting smoking and improving mood in many individuals, according to our evidence. It is also important to note that stopping smoking has not been shown to worsen the health of people with mental illness.

If these findings are confirmed, millions of people unable to quit smoking due to worsening mental health conditions may gain hope.

Individuals may also remain motivated during withdrawal if they are aware that quitting smoking improves mental and social well-being within weeks.

The effects of withdrawal symptoms are temporarily reduced when someone smokes. Smokers must keep up their smoking rate in order to avoid withdrawal symptoms. It is through this phenomenon that nicotine addiction is fueled.

The benefits of smoking, however, are not meaningful or long-term. Smoking and mental health are associated, scientists have found. The general population smokes twice the amount of cigarettes as people with mental health disorders. Scientists need to conduct more research in order to fully understand the relationship between depression and smoking. Previous studies have shown an association between depression and smoking. Nicotine dependence is persistently linked to depression, regardless of age.

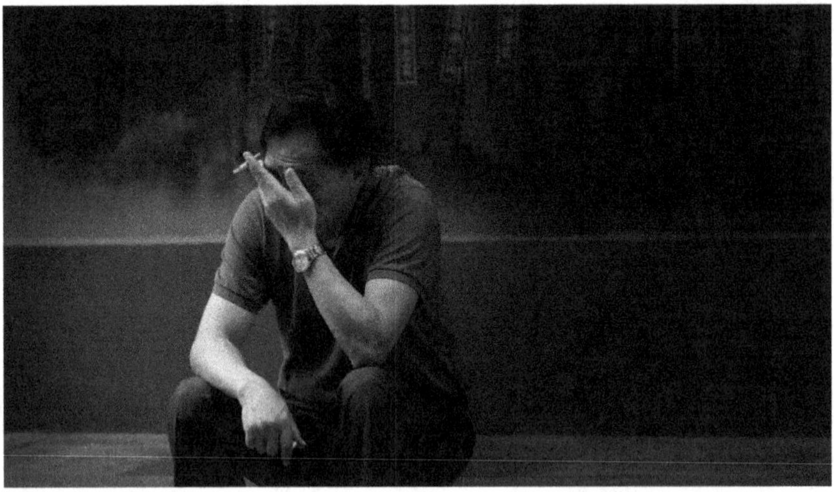

Nicotine and dopamine

When someone inhales smoke, nicotine reaches the brain within 10 to 20 seconds of inhalation. Nicotine is the primary active ingredient in tobacco cigarettes. Once inside, dopamine is released. An important neurotransmitter linked to positive feelings is dopamine. Relaxing your muscles and reducing stress are some of the benefits of this treatment. Relaxation is almost immediate when these properties are present. Nicotine, however, has a short-lived positive impact.

Nicotine's effects

- Tobacco smoke contains nicotine and other synthetic substances that are readily absorbed into the bloodstream through the lungs. Nicotine spreads to every part of the body from that point on.

- Nicotine causes enchanting emotions and distracts the client from unpleasant feelings at the point when taken in limited quantities. Tobacco clients are compelled to use more. The cerebral cortex and the sensory system play a role in influencing temperament in this book. A chemical called dopamine floods the brain's reward circuits when nicotine is ingested, similar to other irresistible medications. Furthermore, nicotine stimulates the adrenal glands - not enough to see, but just enough to raise the heart rate and dilate the vessels.

- After having a drag, nicotine reaches the cerebrum within a few seconds, and its properties begin to fade within minutes. Clients may feel restless and aggravated. In general, withdrawal symptoms are not triggered, but over time, the individual using the item becomes more awkward. Smokers are driven by this to light up once again. The cycle continues until finally the individual uses tobacco, the sentiments disappear, and the cycle continues. Smokers who don't smoke again in a short amount of time can expect their withdrawal symptoms to diminish.

- When the body becomes accustomed to nicotine, individual users will build up the amount of tobacco they use. In turn, their blood contains more nicotine, and this will cause increased rates of nicotine addiction. Resistance is a term used to describe this. The individual should maintain usage to keep up an acceptable level of nicotine over the long haul.

- In the event that a smoker decides to give up smoking, they may experience immediate physical and enthusiastic (mental or mental) withdrawal symptoms. Anxiety, craziness, cerebral pains, and trouble sleeping are some of these manifestations. However, the true hallmark of habit is that individuals will continue to smoke despite knowing it's bad for them - not only affecting their lives, but also affecting those around them. Smokers must halt their habit, in fact.

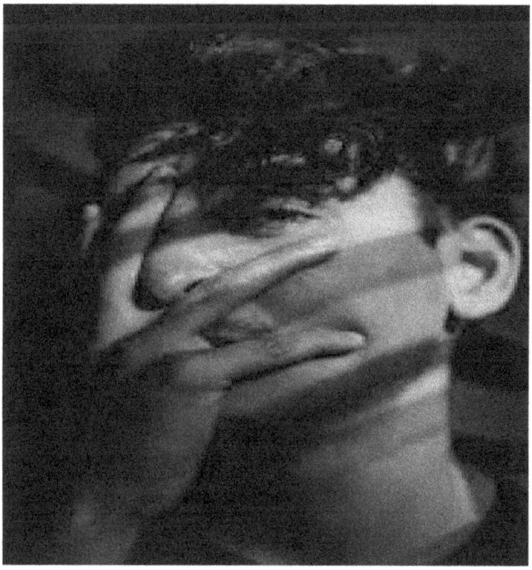

What is the duration of nicotine's stay in the body?

Approximately half of nicotine will be lost after two hours in the body. In other words, nicotine's half-life is 2 hours. Since nicotine has a short half-life, people soon feel as though they need more nicotine.

More than 20 substances are broken down into nicotine, including cotinine, anabases, and nor nicotine, in the body. In urine, these byproducts are ultimately excreted. The following tests can be used by doctors to measure nicotine and nicotine byproducts in a person's system:

- In urination
- Hemoglobin
- Salivation
- hair
- Fingernails

American Association for Clinical Chemistry reports that it may take over 2 weeks for cigarette smokers' blood cotinine levels to equal those of someone who doesn't smoke. The urine levels need to drop for several weeks before they reach very low levels. In research, a hair test is rarely asked for unless people are taking part. However, nicotine traces may stay in hair for longer.

Those who smoke more and smoke more frequently take longer for nicotine takes to leave the body. Nicotine takes different amounts of time to clear depending on the individual:

- People over 65 years of age may be able to absorb nicotine longer.
- When taking birth control pills, most women process nicotine faster than men.
- For people who smoke frequently and for a long time, the body will take longer to remove nicotine.

Nicotine withdrawal lasts how long?

Individuals' level of tobacco use will determine the severity and timing of withdrawal symptoms.

The findings of the study suggest that tobacco users who smoke five or fewer cigarettes daily have less intense physical symptoms. Smoking may still remain an emotional experience for them, however.

In the days to a couple of weeks following smoking, the symptoms of nicotine withdrawal are at their worst. Symptoms usually begin to fade gradually over the course of the week, with the most difficult week being the first.

A person may still feel a psychological desire to smoke even after all physical symptoms have gone away and all nicotine has left their body. The habit of smoking is often the reason for this.

In triggering situations, nicotine desire may be greater. Stress and drinking with friends are suitable examples of these situations. The power of these triggers lessens over time.

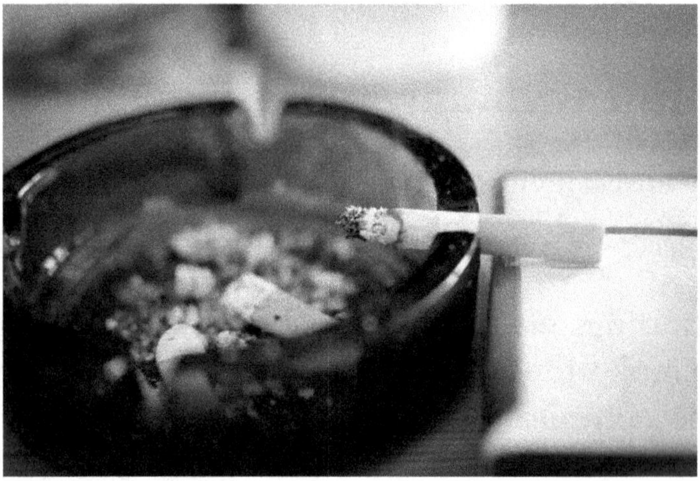

Is it possible to remove nicotine from the body?

- Nicotine can still be detected in blood tests after a period of 10 days if you don't use nicotine for up to ten days before taking the test.
- Nicotine cannot be flushed from the body instantly, but people should maintain a healthy lifestyle so their bodies work efficiently.
- Nicotine can be removed from the body using the following methods:
- Keep your kidneys and liver flushed by drinking plenty of water.
- Sweat releases waste products and gets the blood flowing.
- Ensure that you consume a healthy diet that is high in antioxidants.
- Herbal remedies and commercial products claim to speed the body's ability to clear nicotine from the system, but these products have rarely been adequately tested by regulators.

Physiological, psychological and social effects:

The physiological, psychological, and social effects of nicotine make it harder to quit and fuel your nicotine addiction. The three things can't be separated," Seidman says.

Nicotine's physiological effects

Nicotine triggers the release of adrenaline in your brain once it reaches it. Adrenalin rises when:

- Faster heartbeats
- An increase in your blood pressure
- A quickening of your pulse
- Venous constriction
- Brain activity changes as a result of your environment

There may be some discomfort at first and symptoms such as coughing, headaches, dizziness, or nausea may result. Continuing to smoke, however, will cause these physical changes to become so ingrained that you won't notice them anymore.

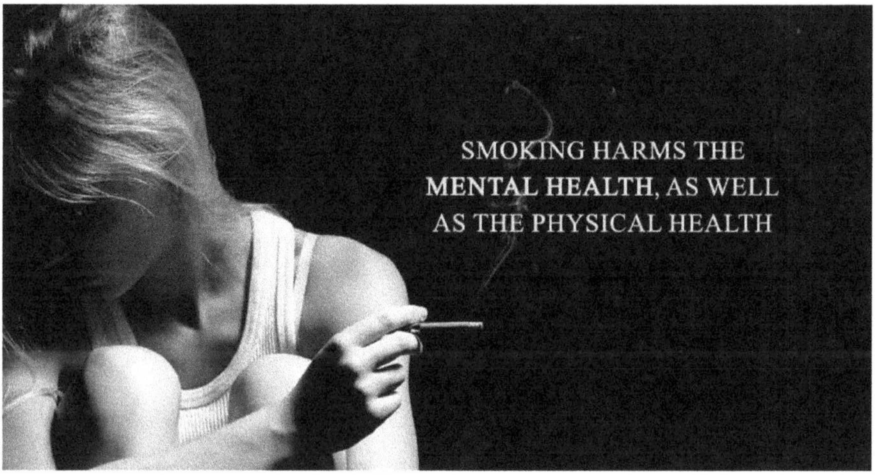
SMOKING HARMS THE
MENTAL HEALTH, AS WELL
AS THE PHYSICAL HEALTH

Nicotine's psychological effects

Nicotine releases excess dopamine in the brain, making you feel relaxed and pleasant. Although the good feeling lasts only a short time, you crave another smoke to continue feeling good.

Using nicotine in cigarettes makes your body more tolerant to its effects. The more cigarettes you smoke, the more you feel relaxed and pleasant, Seidman says. Smoking a pack a day can easily turn into six packs a day, even though it harms your health more as you increase your intake.

Nicotine's social effects

Obtaining, handling, and lighting a cigarette can cause smokers to associate it with pleasure, making their cravings for cigarettes much stronger.

NIDA reports that nearly 60% of young smokers are under the age of 18. As a rebellious act, teens who smoke do so as a way to assert themselves. Teens who smoke may also be influenced by peer pressure. Once they become adults, nicotine has become so addictive they can't stop.

Withdrawal symptoms of nicotine

There is a very real danger of nicotine withdrawal. Because of this, so many smokers attempt to quit more than once before they give up for good.

From hormones to metabolism and the brain, nicotine affects every part of your body. Withdrawal occurs when you no longer possess it. In the absence of nicotine, you will physically crave it.

Although withdrawal from nicotine usually lasts only a month or two, mentally battling cigarettes may last for many months.

As well as physical and mental symptoms, nicotine withdrawal can cause gastrointestinal issues. I always find the first week to be the most difficult, especially the third and fifth days. Eventually, your body will be free of nicotine and you will begin to experience headaches, cravings, and sleep problems. Approximately two weeks after quitting, most people relapse. You will be able to overcome the physical symptoms -- but you will still have stressful mental and emotional challenges like anxiety, depression, and irritability. After a few weeks, they will also decrease.

Withdrawal symptoms on the physical level

Depending on how many cigarettes you smoke every day and how long you have been smoking, you may experience withdrawal symptoms. Health issues in quitting smokers are usually accompanied by these symptoms:

- **Arousal of appetite.**

In the days following your last cigarette, you will experience an increase in appetite. When smokers smoke, their brain releases neurotransmitters such as serotonin and dopamine more rapidly. As a result, you'll eat more when you're not taking these two chemicals. People who used to smoke also find that they eat in order to pass the time while they are doing so. The result will be an increase in cravings for carbs and sweets. People who are trying to quit smoking typically gain 5 to 10 pounds during the first two weeks.

- **Temptations**

In the days following your last cigarette, you could experience nicotine cravings for as long as 30 minutes. Generally, each craving will last for no more than 15 minutes, however there will be other cravings as well. If you want to cope with cravings, you will need to avoid triggers (like alcohol or smoking around others) and find habits that help you cope.

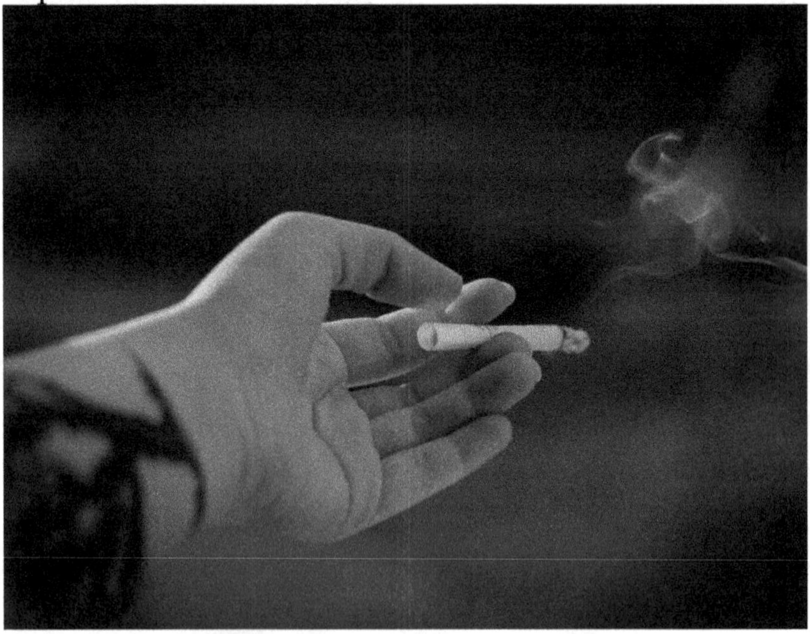

- **Itchy throat**

When nicotine is present, your respiratory system cannot clean itself very well. You may experience a cough before your body works it out.

- **Symptoms include headaches and dizziness.**

This type of withdrawal symptom is generally mild, and it usually comes first and lasts for the first few days.

- **Tiredness**.

You'll probably feel tired without nicotine, since it is a stimulant and wakes you up. However, you may experience restlessness, as well as insomnia.

- **Digestion problems**

One of the unpleasant side effects in the first month is digestion problem.

Nicotine intake management

Tobacco users have a strong tendency to keep their nicotine intake from tobacco within extremely narrow tipping thresholds. They avoid intakes that are either too mild (causing withdrawal) or overly high (causing withdrawal) (resulting in nicotine excess). Nicotine cravings emerge early in the cigarette experience and seem to be consistent throughout time. When switching to cigarettes with less tar and nicotine, admissions decrease owing to nicotine adjustment. The psychological mechanism, compensatory puffing and inward breath, maintains nicotine admissions.

Because nicotine and carbon transportation in smoke are inextricably linked, compensatory smoking also maintains tar admittance and negates any possible health gain from reduced tar cigarettes. Similar compensatory behaviour occurs after reducing the number of cigarettes smoked each day; therefore, this conventional strategy fails to communicate any significant medical benefits.

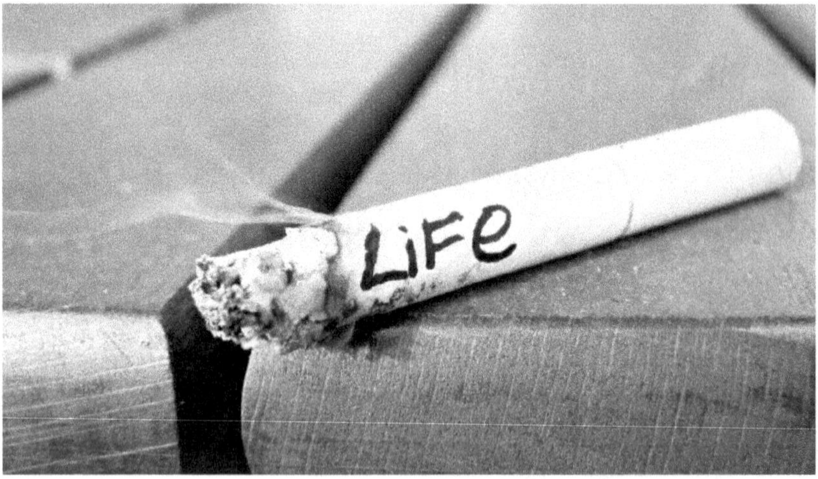

Symptoms relating to the mind, emotions, and behavior

Having quit smoking, you may experience varying degrees of mental and emotional effects. If you are experiencing withdrawal, you may need to deal with some or all of the following:

- **Stress**

The stress that you relieve when you smoke can cause your anxiety to increase. A couple of weeks later, it usually pops up.

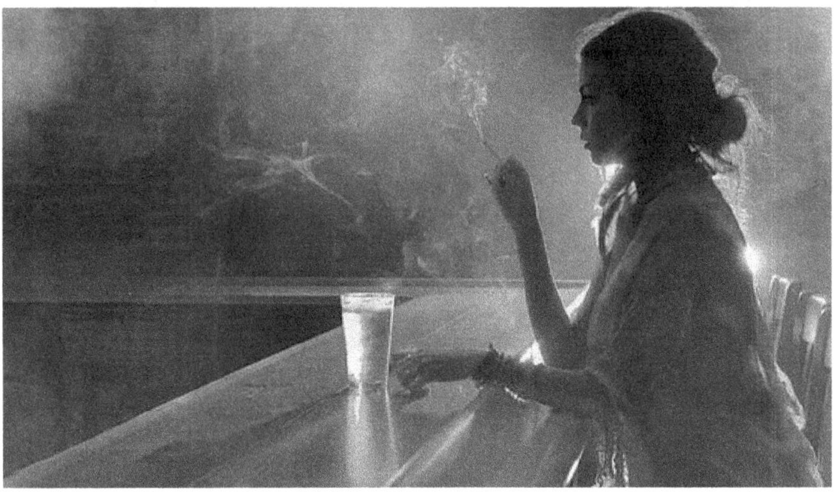

- **mood disorder**

You may start feeling it the day after quitting, but it usually goes away within a month. In the case of anxiety and/or depression, your symptoms may last longer, and you may require additional medical attention.

- **Intolerance**

Managing the physical symptoms may cause you to have a short fuse -- or even make you angry. There's nothing to worry about; it will pass.

- **Fog of mind**

The nicotine will wear off and leave your body as you struggle to concentrate.

The timeline for withdrawing from nicotine

After you smoke your last cigarette, here are some things you can expect:

- Between 30 minutes and 4 hours:

Your nicotine craving will kick in when the effects wear off.

- During the next ten hours:

The time will pass very slowly, and you'll be famished and restless. Feeling down and hopeless can be depressing.

- During the 24 hour period:

An increase in appetite and irritability results.

- Within two days:

The nicotine will leave your body and give you headaches.

- During the third day:

Now that the nicotine is gone, everything should be normal. There will be a decrease in cravings but an increase in anxiety.

- In one week:

It's been a week since you started. Despite the worst, you have survived. Stay away from those triggers.

- Between two and four weeks:

You will still be drained, but you will have more energy and less appetite. You will also feel less anxious, depressed, and cough.

- After 5 weeks:

It is now a matter of staying mentally strong.

Smoking during pregnancy

Smoking during pregnancy raises the chance of:

Pregnancy loss

In addition to bleeding during pregnancy and placental separation, pregnancy complications can also include preterm delivery and ectopic pregnancy.

Weight at birth is low

Smoking mothers have babies who are 200 g (8 oz) lighter on average than mothers without smoking habits. An infant who is premature or underweight is more likely to be sick or infected.

Cleft palates are examples of congenital abnormalities in newborns.

One-third of the risk increases when a baby dies or is stillborn in the first week.

Child's growth, development, and health suffer as a result. Children born to smokers are smaller, have poorer reading and math performance, and are more likely to acquire asthma than children born to nonsmokers.

For additional information, see the Pregnancy and Smoking booklet.

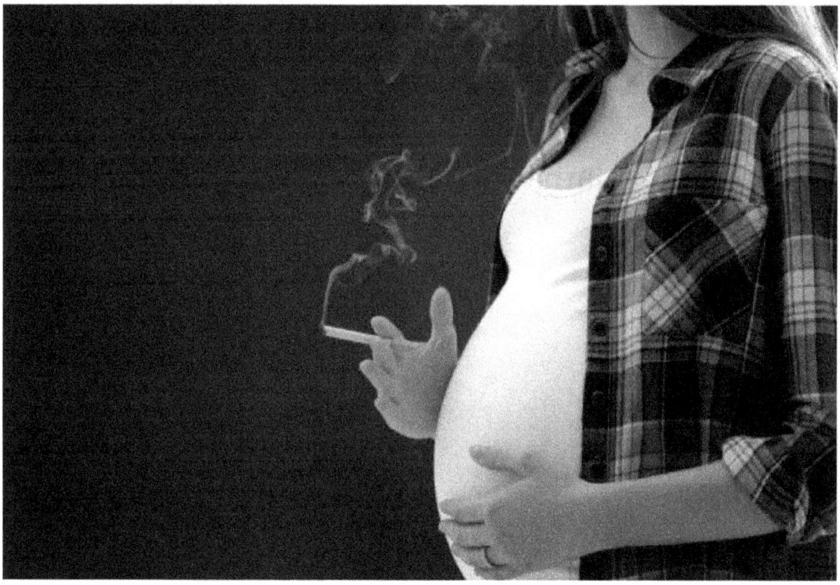

What effect does smoking have on other people?

Your smoke may have an impact on children, nonsmoking adults, and unborn infants.

Children who grow up in a home with a smoker are more likely to suffer from a variety of health issues than children who do not. You don't even have to be smoking in the room or car while a kid is present for your smoke to damage them.

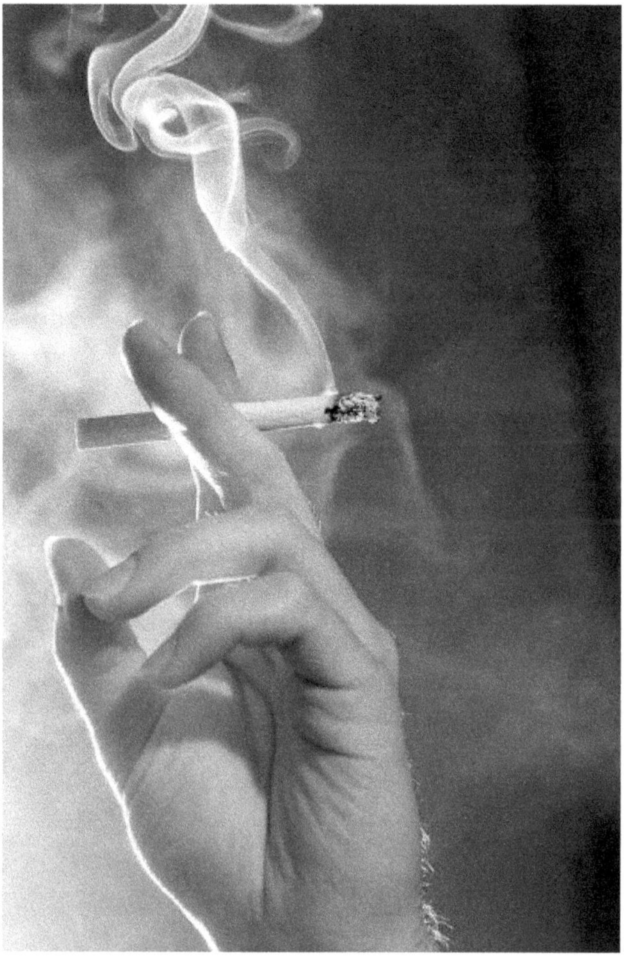

Other drawbacks of smoking

- Stale tobacco pervades your breath, clothing, hair, skin, and house. If you smoke, you don't notice the scent; nevertheless, the stench is noticeable and unpleasant to nonsmokers.
- Your senses of taste and smell have been muted. Food enjoyment may be decreased.
- Cigarette smoking is costly.
- Life insurance is more costly.
- Employers are aware that smokers are more likely than non-smokers to take sick leave, making it more difficult to find work. Each year, more than 34 million working days (1 percent of total) are missed due to tobacco medical leave.
- Potential friendships and relationships may be jeopardized.

Why do women continue to smoke during pregnancy?

According to Livingstone, smoking is more prevalent in some areas than others. Since a high level of deprivation is closely related to socioeconomic factors, it is not surprising that these are areas of very high deprivation."

"The truth is that women face numerous difficulties in their life, and some of them may take precedence," she says. "When people are coping with tough situations, the smoking messages do not reach them. I believe it's critical that we don't blame or condemn women, but they do need to know the facts."

What is the amount of passive smoking that is dangerous?

Passive smoking has a significant impact on health. As a result of the high number of people who are exposed to passive smoking, the health risks of the individual are small compared to active smoking.

The UK Heart Foundation estimates that people living with smokers in their home are 50-60% more likely to die from coronary heart disease. Statistically, it kills 2,700 people between 20 to 64 and 8,000 people between 65 and older each year.

In 2011, children in the UK were estimated to have been visited by 300,000 GPs and admitted to 9,500 hospitals due to inhaling other people's smoke. Second-hand smoke is frequently present in the homes of up to five million children.

In response to a survey, the Department of Health has posted the results on its website. Children want a smoke-free life, according to the survey.

Cigarettes with a variety of flavors

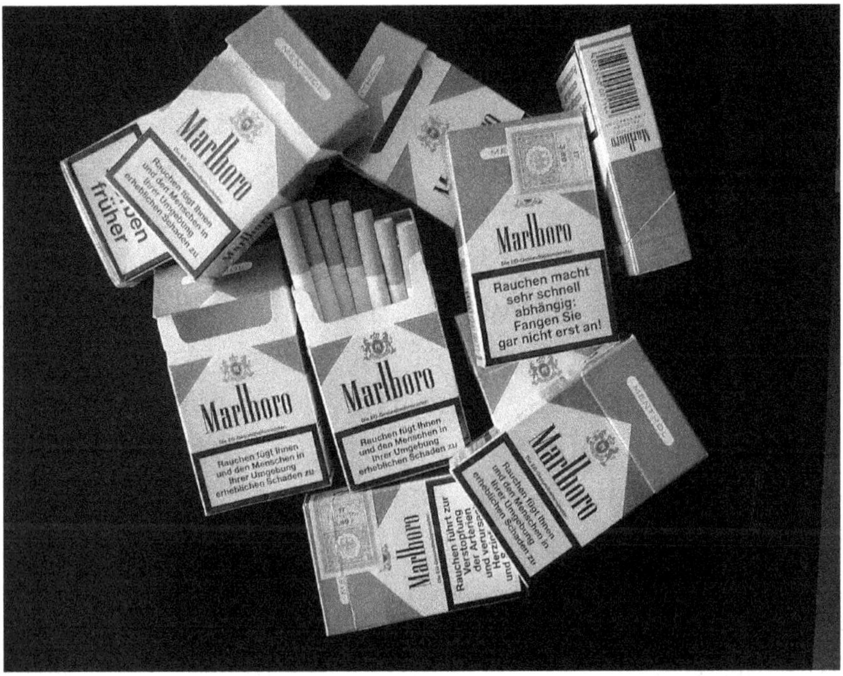

Combination cigarettes do not involve smoking two or more cigarettes simultaneously. This leads to you questioning why you smoked the first one to begin with. The back of my hand was once burned when I put a cigarette into my mouth when I had already put one in. Actually, it isn't nearly as ridiculous as you may believe. As previously said, smoking a cigarette ultimately fails to provide relief from withdrawal symptoms, and even while you are smoking a cigarette, there is still a sense that something is missing. This is the source of a great deal of aggravation for the chain smoker. You are already smoking whenever you need a boost, which is why heavy smokers often resort to alcohol or other substances when they require a boost. But, I digress. A combination cigarette is one that is prompted by two or more of our typical motives for smoking, such as social events, parties, weddings, and meals in restaurants, among others. These are some instances of situations that may be both stressful and soothing at the same time. However, this isn't a contradiction in the traditional sense of the word. Any kind of socialising, especially with friends, can be stressful, and yet you want to be having a good time and feeling totally at ease at the same time you are doing it.

There are instances in which all four of the aforementioned factors are present at the same moment. Driving is one of these activities. Now is a good time to relax if you are leaving a stressful environment, such as a visit to the dentist or the doctor. Driving, on the other hand, usually entails a certain amount of anxiety. It's your life that's on the line. You'll also have to pay attention to what you're doing. Although you may be unaware of the last two variables, the fact that they are subconscious does not rule out the possibility that they are there. Furthermore, if you are delayed in traffic or have a lengthy trip on the highway, you may get bored.

In addition, a game of cards is a famous example. The ability to focus is required while playing games such as bridge or poker. When you are losing more money than you can afford, it may be very distressing. It may get tedious if you go for extended periods of time without receiving a good hand. During this time, you are at leisure and should be resting, which is exactly what you should be doing. All smokers will be chain smoking throughout a game of cards, no matter how minor the withdrawal symptoms are. This includes those who would normally not smoke. In no time, the ashtrays would be completely full and overflowing.

There will be a persistent fall-out fog above the level of the ground. The response you would get if you tapped one of the smokers on the shoulder and asked him whether he was having a good time would be, "You have got to be kidding." It is often after nights like these, when we wake up with a throat that feels like a cess pit, that we make the decision to quit smoking.

This kind of combination cigarette is often one of a kind, and it is typically one of the ones that we believe we would miss the most when we are considering quitting smoking. We believe that life will never be exactly the same pleasure as it was before. However, the same mechanism is at work: these smokes merely offer relief from withdrawal symptoms, and we have a higher desire to alleviate them at certain times of the day than we do at other times of the day.

Let's be very clear about this. It is not the cigarette itself that is noteworthy; rather, it is the occasion. Such times will become more pleasant and difficult circumstances will become less stressful once the desire for a cigarette has been eliminated from the equation

Antidepressants and their role

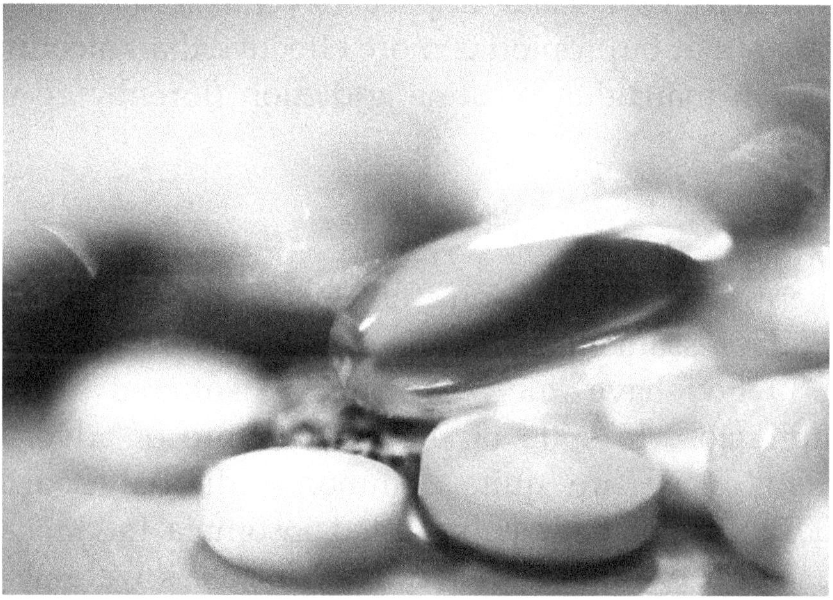

According to Hughes et al. (2001), two reasons exist for why antidepressants can be helpful in quitting smoking.

- First, nicotine withdrawal can trigger depression, and quitting smoking can worsen depression.
- Antidepressants increase dopamine, serotonin, and norepinephrine, which are all involved in smoking.

For the same reasons, some individuals who choose pharmaceutical therapy choose not to take a nicotine replacement while quitting smoking. A systematic study demonstrates the efficacy of two antidepressants, bupropion and nortriptyline (Hughes et al, 2001). According to the researchers, the effects were not clearly unique to particular medicines or a class impact. Several studies have shown that bupropion is more effective than nicotine gum in managing nicotine addiction (Jorenby et al, 1999).

Interestingly, bupropion's efficacy is not due to its antidepressant effect in patients who have depression or who have not previously suffered from depression. In spite of the mild nature of adverse events, they are quite common (Editorial Board, 2001). 40% of patients reported insomnia in clinical trials, for example. Anxiety and dizziness were also reported. Nausea and dry mouth may occur in some patients. The drug has also been linked to severe allergic reactions. An estimated 12 percent of people taking bupropion discontinued treatment after experiencing its adverse effects (Jorenby et al, 1999). According to Hughes et al. (1999), bupropion should not be prescribed to smokers with a history of seizures, anorexia, heavy alcohol use, or head trauma. It is recommended to take bupropion 300mg a day for 7-12 weeks (Hughes et al., 1999). Almost 419,000 people have been prescribed Zyban (bupropion) since it was first licensed in the UK in June 2000. There were 5352 adverse reactions recorded during this time period (BBC News Online,

2001); 37 people have died after taking the drug during this period.

In analyzing adverse reports, the Committee on Safety of Medicine (CSM) determined that less than 1% of them involved a fatal outcome for Zyban. The CSM has deemed it necessary, however, to change the prescribing rules to prevent dosages from being increased on days 1 through 7 following the prescription in order to reinforce safety measures. In addition, the CSM has recommended enhancing warnings to doctors about seizure risks. Coroner's report calls for manufacturers to offer better warnings about mixing it with other medications (BBC News Online, 2001). There is still a lot of room for study and consideration in relation to the most effective use of bupropion for therapeutic purposes (Silagy et al, 2001). A medical intervention involves three possible stages: pre-plan, the change itself, and maintaining the change (Prochaska & Di Clemente, 1983). Behavioral aspects of medicine, especially those related to health promotion, follow this same pattern. Patients can be assisted and encouraged to move through these different stages with the help of their doctors (Goldberg et al., 1994). The assistance and encouragement may lead to some smokers quitting, while others may benefit from referral to a formal smoking intervention program, or simply from continuing surveillance and contact with the doctor's office (Ockene, 1987). There is knowledge, however, that structured behavioral interventions that assist smokers to quit are more effective in assisting them to quit (Walsh & Redman, 1993). In the following text, we will explain how to follow a set of steps during a one-on-one consultation. US clinical practice guidelines (The Agency for Health Care Policy and Research, 1996) provide the foundation for these steps. By setting up follow-up contacts, the approach can be enhanced if both the doctor and the patient are motivated to do so. A doctor should not view the recommended steps (the 5As) as a prescriptive formula, but rather as a basic strategy that can be modified according to clinical circumstances. The 5As can be incorporated into routine healthcare practices in developed and developing nations alike because they are low-cost. Moreover, any intervention aimed at altering health behavior is likely to be more effective if it takes into account the patient's beliefs regarding health and willingness to change.

The stop smoking message is also promoted indirectly in addition to direct patient intervention.

Smoking and tobacco use should be discussed

The problem of smoking should be addressed first and foremost during a medical consultation. Smoking is prominently marked on the patient's agenda, indicating that it is a significant problem. People in poor nations, particularly in certain developing countries, may be ignorant of fundamental health and tobacco facts. The tobacco business may exacerbate the lack of risk knowledge via largely unfettered advertising efforts (Samet & Yoon, 2001). The introduction of the smoking issue may help to justify an organised intervention tailored to the patient. A health practitioner may then integrate the 5As into regular health treatment. You may ask patients whether they are comfortable being questioned about their social habits, such as drinking and smoking. It is critical to educate patients who have tobacco-related symptoms that their difficulties are the result of tobacco usage and that they should think about quitting. Patients who do not have tobacco-related symptoms will need to have a broad conversation about cigarette use. At this point, the health practitioner may stress that quitting smoking is arguably the most essential action that can be done to preserve one's health after basic needs such as food, clothes, housing, and employment are fulfilled, as well as the absence of contagious illnesses.

Smoking status should be assessed

A standard general process should include periodic evaluations of tobacco use. Whether or not a patient has ever smoked and how much they usually smoke should be asked of every patient each year after high school: "Are you a smoker?" Not only should patients with smoking-related symptoms be questioned, but so should all patients. It is recommended that patients who claim to have recently stopped smoking be questioned whether they still smoke on occasion, since deception rates seem to be greater in this population (Nagle, 1996). The smoking status of patients should be fully documented in the medical record, as should their alcohol use. Smokers should also be questioned about their smoking history, including how long they have been smoking and if they have made any prior efforts to quit. Non-smokers, particularly former smokers, should be congratulated on their decision to abstain from smoking.

Provide advice on quitting smoking and determine the patient's willingness to do so

Examine to see whether the patient is thinking about quitting and counsel him or her appropriately. "Have you considered quitting smoking?" If the patient is not interested in quitting, encourage him or her to do so by pointing out that the patient's present sickness or health issues may be linked to smoking.

- Strategies for patient motivation should concentrate on health issues specific to the particular patient, as well as the advantages of quitting. As shown in Table 1, provide your individual reasons for leaving.
- Make it quite clear you are concerned, for example, "As a doctor, I am concerned that you smoke; it would be better if you quit."
- Inquire with the patient about the dangers of smoking and the advantages of stopping. Correct incorrect ideas and reinforce appropriate ones. Analogies between the effects of nicotine, tar, and carbon monoxide may aid in explaining the major dangers. If this is a problem for the patient, specifically refute the tobacco industry's claims that "low tar" cigarettes are safer than normal smokes (Bates et al, 1999). Table 2 lists some of the most

frequent reasons patients offer for not giving up, as well as acceptable answers for the clinician.

- Educate patients on the dangers of passive smoking and appeal to their feeling of responsibility.
- Inform the patient that assistance is available if he or she is ready later. Mention referral agencies.
- If you have access to resources, provide literature and film/videos on the dangers of smoking.

Patients who are ready to quit, or who have already started quitting, may need assistance

Doing the following will help you reinforce the decision to stop: You may be doing the best thing for your long-term health by doing that.

- If the patient is still smoking, negotiate a quit date and note it in the medical record. Patients who establish a specific deadline are more likely to make a genuine effort (Cummings et al, 1986). The appointment should be scheduled quickly, and for many patients, there is no better time than the day of their medical consultation. Some patients may want to select a different time (ideally within 7 days) that is more convenient for them.
- Emphasize the significance of going "cold turkey." As previously stated, gradual decrease seldom leads to cessation on its own.
- Address typical issues that patients anticipate, such as withdrawal symptoms, weight gain, stress, social pressure, and recurrence. Table 3 contains strategies for coping with typical issues.

- Encourage the patient to provide recommendations based on their own experience to assist them in quitting smoking. Previous efforts may be viewed as preparation for effectively quitting. Table 4 contains a collection of halting suggestions.
- Instruct on behavioral skills, such as alternative behavior or relaxation techniques.
- If necessary, prescribe NRT or bupropion (see pages 14-16). Motivated, but more addicted, individuals may benefit from NRT; nevertheless, NRT with clear use instructions must be used in conjunction with cessation counseling. Table 11 outlines the patient instructions for NRT.
- Explain why NRT is necessary: For example, "Nicotine replacement treatment is not a miracle cure." It will, however, help you manage with the withdrawal symptoms and cravings involved with quitting, as well as giving you time to focus on issues such as dealing with stress or boredom."
- Offer self-help resources in addition to your advice.
- Arrange for a follow-up Examine the patient's development and provide encouragement and reinforcement as needed. Relapse prevention, such as addressing how the patient will cope with smoking signals, is an essential component

of any behavior modification programmed. For example, if the patient usually smokes with a cup of coffee or after a meal, he or she should be urged to alter this pattern in order to avoid this set of signals to smoke. Reassure patients who have relapsed, investigate what went wrong, and encourage them to try again. If NRT or bupropion has been prescribed, follow-up contacts allow dosage, promote compliance, and allow the length of usage to be tracked.

Dealing with common problems: strategies

Problem No. 1 -

You may suffer withdrawal symptoms if you stop smoking. They usually appear within 24 hours after quitting, peak about three days later, and gradually decrease over the next three weeks. It may take more than three months to become accustomed to not smoking.

These symptoms may manifest themselves both physically and psychologically:

- Mouth dryness, painful throat, gums, or tongue (coping: drink water, fruit juice, chew gum)

- Headache, forehead tightness, muscle spasms, leg spasms, and leg cramps (coping: take a warm bath or shower, try relaxation or meditation)

- Anger, tenseness, anxiety, decreased attention span, headache, tachycardia (coping: take a walk, take a bath or shower, try relaxation or meditation)

Appetite grows.

(As a coping strategy, drink water or low-calorie beverages and consume low-fat, low-calorie snacks.)

- Abnormalities in bowel motions (coping: add roughage to the diet, e.g. raw fruits and vegetables, drink water)

- Insomnia (coping: avoid caffeinated drinks, calm, and meditate)

- Sleep deprivation (coping: take a nap, relax)

- Coughing fits - natural clearing mechanism (coping: sip warm herbal tea, take cough drops) It is important to reassure patients that side effects are just brief. Only the desire to inhale and an increased hunger may last for a long time (US Department of Health and Human Services, 1990). Patients who are very concerned about addiction should be advised to use NRT.

Gaining Weight Is a Problem No. 2 Smoking seems to reduce calorie efficiency levels and/or increase respiration rate.

Despite the fact that four-fifths of smokers who stop gain weight after quitting, the normal weight increase is just 2.3 kg.

- Emphasize that the health advantages of stopping smoking outweigh the dangers of typical gaining weight.

- Encourage moderate activity, water consumption, avoiding excess calories, sugar free gum, and mixed fruit snacks.

- If the patient finds it hard to follow the above recommendations and stop smoking at the same time, suggest a two-step strategy: First, the patient should abstain from cigarettes while allowing the weight to build; second, after the habit is broken, he or she should concentrate on reducing weight.

Common problems and strategies to solve them (continued)

Stress is the third issue.

To deal with stress, many patients smoke.

• Suggest basic relaxation techniques, such as "take a calm, deep breath and, as you breathe out, repeat to yourself "relax." Do this ten times."

• Distribute a stress-relief booklet or link to a relaxation class. See Module Preparation for Invasive Procedures for further information.

4th Issue - Social Pressure

• Dealing with offers of cigarettes from other smokers may be difficult. The patient should practice expressing "no" emphatically.

• If there is a high danger of relapse, alcohol drinking circumstances should be avoided for a short period of time.

• Patients who are worried about previous failed efforts to quit should be reassured that most smokers achieve long-term cessation only after many tries. Slipping is completely natural and should not deter people from continuing with their current attempts to quit. Previous efforts should be regarded as useful practice.

• Remind the patients of their original reason(s) for stopping.

• Talk with the patients about how they can deal with circumstances that have previously been linked to relapse, such as the Five Ds.

Tips for quitting smoking

Information for patients regarding nicotine replacement therapy

Individualize these suggestions for each patient. Suggestions include the following:

• The Five Ds are abbreviated as "The Five Ds." Patients may find it beneficial to recall and practice the Five Ds.

When faced with the desire to smoke:

- Delay, even if only for a brief time

- Drink plenty of water.

- Deep inhalation

- Try something new and

- Talk about the desire with another person; • make a list of reasons to stop and post it publicly, such as on the fridge.

• Remove all tobacco items, ashtrays, lighters, matches, and so forth from all places in which you live.

• Clean all clothing to eliminate cigarette odours; • Enlist the help of nonsmoking friends, family, and coworkers; and • Modify smoking behaviors, such as chewing on a toothpick or changing rooms instead of smoking after meals.

To avoid a reflex reaction to smoke while talking on the phone, move the phone to a different location.

• Maintain a daily routine to minimize association of tobacco with certain activities or times of day • Sit in non-smoking areas • Avoid situations that could lead to relapse, e.g. go to the bathroom • deep breathe • positive self-talk

You can say "No thanks, I don't smoke"; suggest that other smokers don't provide cigarettes or offer to purchase cigarettes; recall why you stopped smoking in the first place; and see quitting as a process rather than an instant lifetime commitment.

In general, nicotine replacement therapy is not a miracle cure. It may help you deal with withdrawal symptoms, but it does not provide the same amount of nicotine as cigarettes.

· To quit smoking for good, you'll still need to put in a lot of effort.

After 1-2 months, you may start tapering off the medicine; nevertheless, you must not smoke even one puff while taking the drug.

Nicotine chewing gum

1. Take x* doses each waking hour.

2. Do not use as a chewing gum substitute? Compress the gum with your teeth a few times before allowing it to settle in your mouth. Every minute or so, repeat the cycle.

3. Avoid chewing too fast.

4. After approximately 30 minutes, discard the gum.

5. Do not chew gum while drinking.

6. It may take up to a week to become accustomed to the taste of the gum.

Nicotine transdermal

1. Select a hairless location that is suitable for normal clothes.

2. Alter the location every day to minimise the risk of skin irritation.

3. Avoid areas where there has been skin inflammation.

* Dose will be determined following evaluation, although it is usually one dose every waking hour.

Motivating interventions

The last element of intervention that is important to understand and implement is the idea of "motivational interviewing." This approach is founded on the assumption that most patients do not come to you prepared to alter their behaviours, even if it would make you feel better if they did. As a result, even if you attempt to offer them advise on what they should and should not do, you may only have limited success in convincing them to change. In fact, the advice-giving method may actually elicit opposition from them.

A significant portion of the interview consists of affirmation, support, and diplomatic statements. Encourage your patients to express and examine their feelings about their behaviour and change, both for and against it. Before you do anything, ask them how they feel about you bringing up problems, addressing these topics, advising or informing them. When you meet resistance from a patient, halt immediately and take a step backward. If you irritate your patients, they will be considerably less open to your recommendations, and you will become unproductive. During this process, you attempt to gradually move people closer to change. It may take many visits to persuade your patient to change.

Knowing this ahead of time may make it simpler to handle.

Techniques for improving patient memory of information People remember better when they deduce problems for themselves rather than being told; for example, patients should be asked what they believe to be the dangers of continuing to smoke and what they perceive to be the advantages of quitting.

People are more inclined to recall and discuss what is important to them.

There are additional strategies that a doctor can employ to ensure that a patient understands and remembers information.

In every consultation, the following strategies should be used:

• Keep information basic, straightforward, and to the point.

• Avoid technical jargon and provide extra information in layman's terms.

• Speak clearly and slowly. Be mindful that many elderly individuals may have hearing loss.

• Arrange your suggestions into categories. Go through each set one at a time.

- Reiterate critical facts.
- Emphasize the significance of your suggestion.
- Make use of basic diagrams or models.
- Write down or have the patient write out the most essential instructions.
- Make self-help resources available for the patient to take home.
- Summarize the facts at the conclusion of the consultation.
- Assess the patient's comprehension.
- Check to see if there are any lingering questions.

1992 (Professional Education and Training Committee and Postgraduate Medical Council of NSW).

Guidelines for medical educators on how to teach cognitive-behavioral treatments to patients to help them quit smoking

In medical education, smoking has long been under-emphasized as a health concern (Ginzel, 1985). To increase their involvement in smoking intervention, doctors must get sufficient training in preventative counselling skills (Ockene, 1987). To be successful in dealing with a problem as complicated and pervasive as cigarette smoking, physicians must get acquainted with the societal forces involved with smoking and have the motivation, attitude, and abilities to intervene (Ginzel, 1985).

The first step is to educate physicians on the dangers of smoking as a cause of illness. However, a more serious issue is a lack of knowledge regarding smoking cessation methods (Fowler, 1993). Training physicians in these methods may improve the chance that they will advise their patients to quit smoking (Kottke et al., 1989). Medical education on smoking, on the other hand, should not be limited to a single lecture or workshop, but should be incorporated throughout the medical program and experiential learning. The emphasis in the early years of medical school may be primarily on public health and clinicopathological problems, with the emphasis changing in the last years to how physicians may assist smokers quit smoking.

A suggested guidebook for educating medical students about tobacco is also available in addition to the information in this module (Richmond & Songmei, 1998).

Purpose

This training programme outlines the techniques for teaching medical students the skills required for successful interventions to assist people quit smoking.

The resources

• A written learning module that summarises the health hazards of smoking and describes the concepts and techniques of cognitive-behavioral and pharmaceutical treatments for smoking cessation. This criterion may be met by using the first two parts of this learning programme.

• It is recommended that each medical school create a film in which students may see a competent doctor counsel a smoking patient about quitting. This should serve as an example for pupils to build their own approach on. If videotape manufacturing is not a viable option, an audio-tape demonstration would offer an alternative, although less effective, teaching resource.

Alternatively, the authors of this module may provide an English language film of a medical smoking cessation intervention.

• Students should have access to a collection of publications detailing scientific studies and different smoking cessation programmers. The reference list for this module includes important information.

• Each institution should create a set of case scenarios that may be utilized as the foundation for student practice. These should ideally include male and female patients in the different medical settings where smokers may be met, such as community and hospital primary care clinics, obstetric practice, and hospital surgical and medical wards. It would be beneficial to include patients of different ages who have and have not had smoking-related illnesses. Appendix 1 includes two example case situations with recommendations for both the patient and the clinician.

• A rating scale that may be used to evaluate student success in the practice of smoking cessation treatments'.

The procedure

• Students should read the available learning module.

• The students should watch one or two filmed instances of a doctor conducting a smoking cessation intervention; alternatively, an experienced doctor may provide a demonstration using a'simulated patient.' Following the demonstration, students should be given enough time to discuss the interaction(s) they saw.

• A course instructor should walk students through the learning module to ensure they grasp the procedure.

Unless students are also unsure about the dangers of smoking, the emphasis should be on the stages of the intervention component. To demonstrate the suggested procedures, a series of overhead transparencies or slides should be created for use in this session.

• Students should practise the skills needed for a successful intervention.

There are many options for how things may go. If time allows, students may focus on one stage at a time, such as educating about the dangers, fighting self-exemptions, and negotiating a stop date.

The difficulties of properly administering nicotine replacement therapy adequate prior assessment need a distinct emphasis. Alternatively, a whole intervention may be role-played in a single sequence utilising case scenarios from their curriculum. Allow for up to 20 minutes for this reason. Although an experienced clinician may be able to conduct a smoking cessation interview more quickly, students should be given more time to practise the entire repertoire of skills for the first time.

• Where videotape facilities are available, each student can create a videotape in which he or she plays the role of a doctor. Segments of each student's videotape can then be viewed in a tutorial with 4-8 students led by a tutor, and appropriate feedback can be given. Instead of students, 'simulated patients' could be used to play the role of the patient. When there are no videotape facilities available, students can be divided into small groups of 3-5 students, with each student having the opportunity to play the doctor and patient while the other(s) observe and rate the 'performance.' During these sessions, both the tutor and the students should strive to provide constructive feedback.

- A barrier evaluation should be included, in which students must demonstrate acceptable performance in smoking cessation treatments using an objective rating instrument (see Appendix 2). Medical students are more inclined to take learning areas that are thoroughly evaluated seriously.

Behavior Therapy

The behavioral therapies provided by quitting smoking experts are often scheduled for four to eight weeks in duration. For patients, it has been shown that in-person counseling combined with smoking cessation medicines is effective. It is possible to get help in quitting smoking in a variety of ways.

❖ Behavioral Cognitive Therapy:

(CBT) is a kind of therapy in which the patient uses his or her thoughts to solve problems (CBT). The use of cognitive behavioral therapy (CBT) helps the patients recognize trigger points people, areas, and things that cause them to engage in harmful behavior—and means teaching them relapse-prevention skills (such as breathing exercises) and system set strategies to help them avoid smoking when confronted with stressful conditions and triggers. According to the findings of a research that compared cognitive behavioral therapy with basic health education, both treatments decreased nicotine dependency. The results of a separate research showed that patients who engaged in six sessions of intense group cognitive behavioral therapy (CBT) had higher quit rates than patients who engaged in six sessions of overall health education.

❖ Motivational Interviewing

(MI) is a technique that helps people become more motivated (MI)

In MI, counselors assist patients in exploring and resolving their ambiguity about quitting smoking, as well as enhancing their desire to adopt healthy lifestyle modifications. Providers point out differences between patients' objectives or beliefs and their present actions in a non confrontational manner. MI is patient-centered and non confrontational. They make adjustments to accommodate patients' reluctance to change while also encouraging self-efficacy and hope. Studies of MI have shown that this intervention resulted in greater quit rates than either short smoking cessation counseling or standard treatment, according to the findings.

❖ Mindfulness

Meditation assists patients in becoming aware of their thoughts, feelings, desires that could lead to relapse. The patient is taught techniques to cope with negative emotions without giving in to cravings or using tobacco. Stress and cravings are handled without the patients resorting to things such as tobacco or other unhealthy behaviours. During the last decade, there has been a rise in interest in mindfulness-based therapies, and studies have shown that this approach is beneficial to general mental health and may help avoid return to smoking. Clinical studies, on the other hand, must be closely monitored

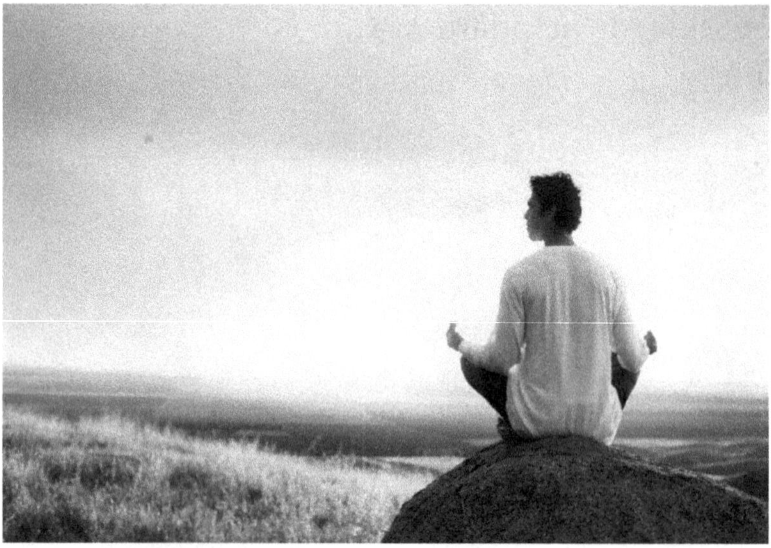

Best tips to stop smoking

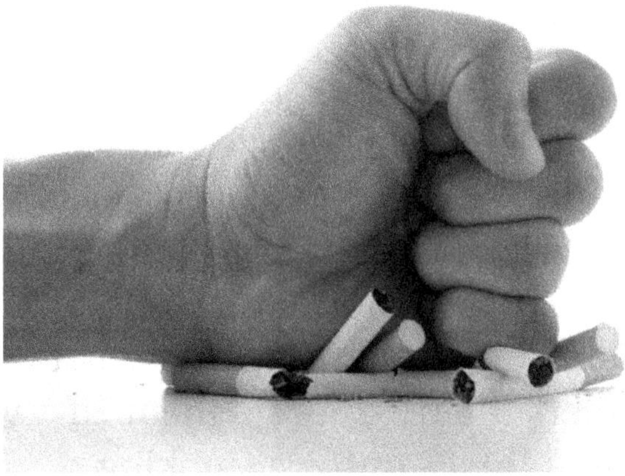

Here is the list of best tips to stop smoking:

1. Keep in mind that the most difficult aspect of quitting is typically the first several days. Mentally prepare yourself to endure just the first two days, then the first week, and you'll be in excellent condition after that. Your body will be detoxing heavily over the first few days, and if you can get through that, you can get through anything
2. Get going. Physical exercise may help reduce nicotine cravings and alleviate certain withdrawal symptoms. Instead of reaching for a cigarette, go for a jog. Even little activity, such as picking weeds in the garden or going for a leisurely walk, may be beneficial. Furthermore,

the increased exercise will burn additional calories and help you avoid weight gain while you stop smoking.

3. if you have a friend or loved one who is struggling to stop smoking, you should try sharing some of the unpleasant facts about smoking with them. Try to be genuine and kind when you relay this information to them so that they understand you are attempting to assist them rather than attack them.2If you're attempting to quit smoking, avoid circumstances or locations that may entice you to smoke. If you've always smoked at happy hour or with your coffee, consider altering your habit. Drinking coffee in the vehicle on your way to work, or finding a new hangout other than the pub, can allow you to reduce typical triggers and cravings.
4. Do not empty your ashtrays. You will be less inclined to smoke if you see how many cigarettes you have smoked in the ashtray. This will also remove the unattractive butts and their odour. This may be useful since it will remind you of how terrible the smoke smell is.
5. You must use caution if you are attempting to stop using crutches such as patches and medication. When you start using these other drugs, you put yourself at risk of developing a

new hazardous addiction. When you first start using your quitting crutches, be cautious.

6. Keep in mind that mindset is important. You must constantly have a good attitude when it comes to quitting smoking. Consider all of the support and assistance you are providing to your body, as well as how much healthier you will be as a result of taking this important step in your life.
7. 265. Anyone attempting to quit smoking should get rid of everything that reminds them of smoking. Remove all ashtrays and lighters from your house. To eliminate the odour of smoke, clean your carpets, draperies, and furniture, as well as your linens, towels, and clothes. These actions will reduce the likelihood that you will be reminded of smoking and develop a cigarette desire.
8. 2If you want to stop smoking cold turkey, get rid of everything that reminds you of smoking in your home. This implies there will be no more ashtrays or cigarette lighters. If you keep this material, it will just remind you of smoking and may make you want to smoke.
9. If you've chosen to quit smoking, psychologically prepare yourself for what's to come. Concentrate on the idea that you have the ability to quit and that this is not an unattainable goal. Set a firm "quit date" and consider putting it on your calendar. Your

chances of quitting will improve if you take such a positive attitude.

10. Always keep in mind that your mindset is everything. When you're starting to feel depressed, try to make yourself proud that you're quitting. Smoking is harmful for you, and each time you overcome the desire to smoke, you should be happy of yourself because you are taking important steps toward a healthier you.
11. When user starts any smoking cessation strategy, make a customized list of actions you may do to quit. Take the time to personalize your list to help you stop smoking more successfully. What works for one person may not work for another. It's critical that you find out which methods work best for you. Making a list of your own techniques can assist you in reaching your objective.

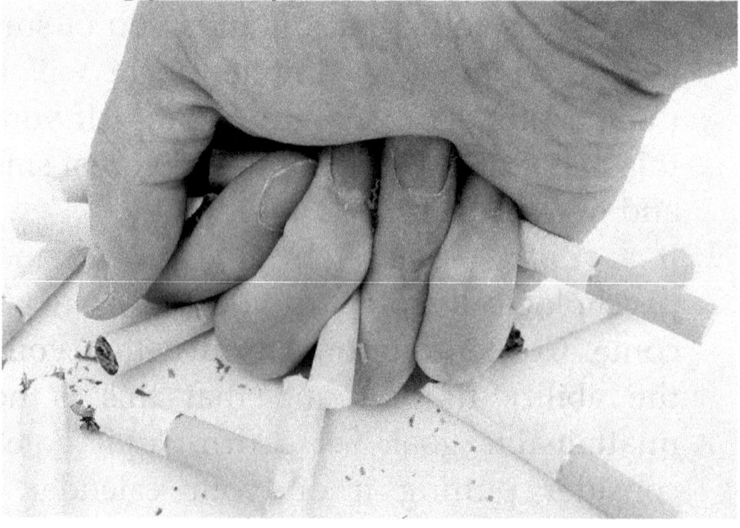

12. When attempting to quit smoking, make a list of all the reasons why you want to quit. Keep a copy of the list with you at all times. One of the greatest places to keep this list is in the same location you used to keep your smokes. Whenever you find yourself reaching for a pack of cigarettes, take out the list and read about why you want to quit smoking.

13. If you plan to stop smoking, you must first discover the reasons that will inspire you to do so. There are compelling reasons to exercise, including safeguarding your family and preventing lung cancer. Respect for your body and for the gift of life is another strong motivator. Whatever excuse you pick, it must be sufficient to keep you from lighting up again in the future Discuss prescription medications with your doctor. Consider prescription medicines to alleviate nicotine withdrawal symptoms. Certain medicines may help decrease cravings by affecting the chemical balance in your brain. There are other medications that may alleviate unpleasant

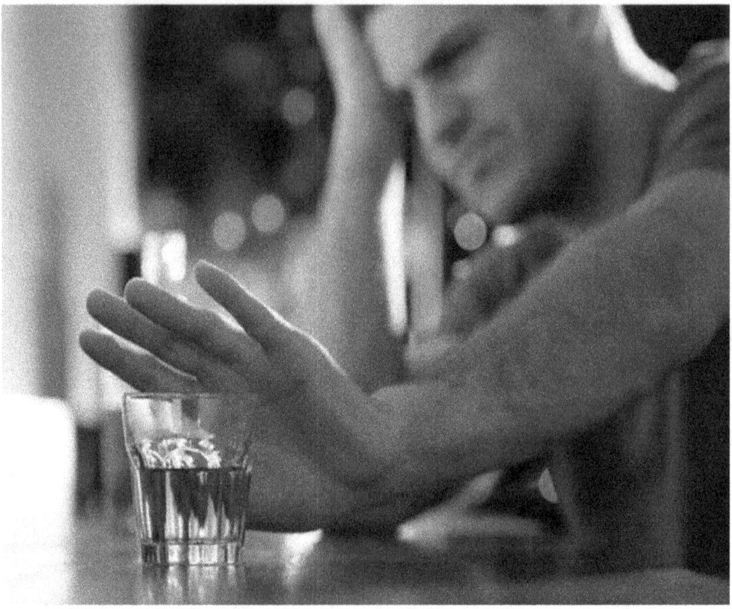

withdrawal symptoms such as difficulty to focus or sadness.

14. Avoid alcohol and other substances that make you want to smoke. Avoiding alcohol and coffee is a recognized smoking trigger, so avoid them if at all feasible. Also, smokers prefer to light up after eating, so do something else, such as washing the dishes or brushing your teeth. 274. Inform everyone you know that you're leaving! They will be there for you whenever you need them and will be able to remind you of your intention to stop. It is important to use a decent support system while quitting. This significantly improves your chances of success and will bring you where you want to go.
15. To avoid blowing smoke, blow off some steam. Exercising is one of the most effective methods to combat nicotine cravings. As an additional

benefit, if you supplement quitting smoking with a more intense exercise regimen, you will feel the results of your improved health more quickly.

16. To keep yourself motivated to stop smoking for good, use the money you save to treat yourself. Calculate how much money you will save by quitting ahead of time, and deposit the money you would have spent on cigarettes in a separate account. When you achieve a small objective, use the money to treat yourself to something pleasant.
17. Don't try to stop smoking if you want to. Quitting smoking is a two-word phrase that implies loss, making it a mourning process. Instead, embrace tobacco-freedom on a psychological level. Think about what would make you happy if you were free of cigarettes, not what would make anybody else happy. What would you be able to accomplish with that money and time? Consider any treatment that can be used to replace nicotine. Smoking is unpleasant and simple to stop, but nicotine withdrawal is typically the last nail in the coffin of a quit attempt. Do all you can to alleviate the withdrawal symptoms, from medication to alternative treatments like as patches, gum, or throat lozenges?
18. Seek help from internet forums and support groups. There are many organizations that are open to everyone or concentrate on a specific

topic. Sharing your quitting difficulties and triumphs with people who understand your struggle may be beneficial or even therapeutic. Other ex-smokers understand your difficulties and the emotional issues that may impede stopping smoking.

19. You must use caution if you are attempting to stop using crutches such as patches and medication. When you start using these other drugs, you put yourself at risk of developing a new hazardous addiction. When you first start using your quitting crutches, be cautious.
20. If you want to stop smoking, don't try to do it overnight. Nicotine addiction is strong, and it will take some time to wean yourself off of it. If you stop cold turkey, you are far more likely to relapse, so go slowly and do it properly the first time.
21. Write out the advantages of smoking cessation to boost your motivation and get smokes out of your everyday routine. Putting things down in paper may change your whole perspective. This may help you remain motivated and may make it easier to stop.
22. Reward yourself if you're succeeding in your quit smoking quest. When you've cut down, reward yourself with a massage, a manicure, or a beautiful new dress, and then do something different when you've completely quit. You need to have incentives like these to look forward to in order to stay motivated.

23. Always have a cool glass or bottle of ice water handy. When you have a cigarette desire, take a drink of water—even if it means putting the bottle down. This offers you something to do with your hands and mouth, and it may also help you avoid eating.
24. Get into a fitness regimen by joining a gym and substituting healthy activity for smoking time. Exercise may help to alleviate the tension caused by nicotine withdrawal. If you don't exercise frequently, start slowly by going for a stroll once or twice a day. Before beginning any fitness programme, consult with your doctor.
25. Be aware of regular actions that stimulate a desire to smoke. It is the first cup of coffee in the morning for some. Others may be at the conclusion of a meal or mingling with smoking buddies. Whatever your trigger is, now is the moment to remind yourself that you are quitting because you care about yourself enough to want to.
26. Exercise, believe it or not, may be the key to quitting smoking. Many individuals smoke because they are overwhelmed or worried. They resort to smokes for comfort when they are anxious. Exercising may be used in lieu of smoking. Exercise is also beneficial to a person's general health.
27. Many people believe that electronic cigarettes are an excellent method to stop smoking. They do not have as many of the harmful

consequences of regular cigarettes and may be an excellent method to gradually reduce your smoking from normal levels to a lower level until you no longer smoke at all.

28. Make a firm commitment to stopping. Individuals who are able to effectively stop smoking devote completely to the process. They don't have a backup plan, they don't keep their decision to resign hidden, and they don't warn themselves that they will fail. If you make this kind of commitment, you will greatly improve your odds of reaching your objective.
29. The most effective method to quit smoking is to stop altogether. The only way to really quit is to stop altogether. Simply attempt to quit smoking and never take up another cigarette again. This technique of stopping smoking is not the simplest. This technique has been proven to be very successful.

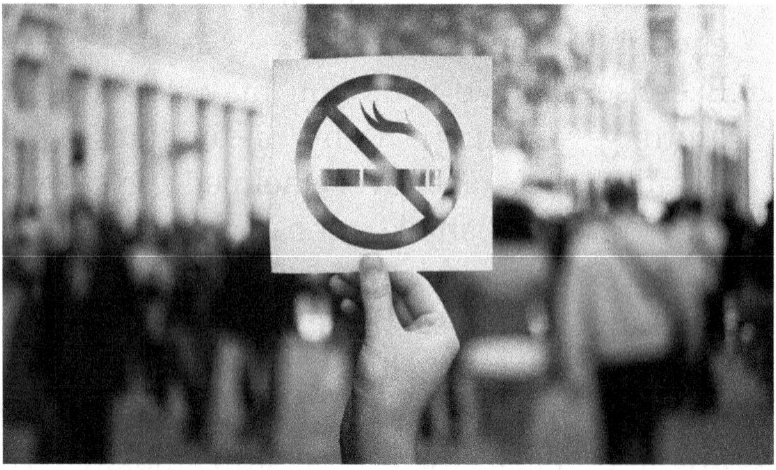

30. Although one of the primary reasons for quitting smoking is to save money, you should treat yourself to a treat now and then with the money you have saved by not smoking.
31. Although one of the primary reasons for quitting smoking is to save money, you should treat yourself to a treat now and then with the money you have saved by not smoking. These joys provide you with something to look forward to while also serving as a reminder of the things you couldn't afford while you were a tobacco user. It is essential that you have a proper incentive structure in place for such a difficult task.
32. It is essential that you have a proper incentive structure in place for such a difficult task . You should give yourself a break for at least the first three days and the first two weeks after you quit using tobacco. Following that, you should commemorate monthly milestones until you reach the annual mark of achievement. You may even be able to customise your reward based on the length of time that has passed, making success extra sweeter.
33. Having a cigarette is a common trigger for many smokers. These triggers may include feeling nervous, completing a meal, or being in a certain location. If you're trying to quit smoking, try to stay away from these triggers as much as possible. If you are unable to

prevent them, devise a strategy to redirect your attention away from the need to smoke.

34. Create a slogan for yourself that says "NOPE, not a single puff, ever." It is possible to convince yourself that one cigarette would not damage you, yet doing so may undo years of hard work and dedication. Take, for example, the potency of a single puff.
35. During the first three days, be sure to drink lots of cranberry juice. Any use of acidic fruit juices can help to alleviate the discomfort of nicotine withdrawal while your body chemistry adapts to the new situation. It is important to remember to quit after three days since the physical effects of nicotine withdrawal will have gone by that time and the juices will just serve to make you fatter.
36. Incorporate regular exercise into your daily routine if you're trying to stop smoking. Physical activity may be beneficial in coping with the nicotine cravings that will inevitably occur after quitting smoking. Physical activity may be beneficial in reducing withdrawal symptoms. If you take a walk with your dog or spend time in your garden, you will find it easier to quit smoking sooner.
37. Being honest with oneself is essential while attempting to quit smoking. Cigarette addiction is a legitimate medical condition, just like any other substance addiction. In order to successfully quit smoking, you need seek both

mental and physical support. Additionally, this suggests that quitting smoking should be a one-and-done proposition.

38. Put out an effort to choose a date for quitting.
39. Put out an effort to choose a date for quitting. Set your quit date far enough in advance so that you have time to prepare, but not so far in advance that it becomes ethereal or impossible to remember. Decide on a day that is not going to be busy or stressful, and mark the date on your calendar so that you may make arrangements ahead of time.
40. Consider quitting smoking cold turkey if you're trying to quit smoking for good. The most convenient method in the long run is to choose the first option. Initially, this may seem to be more difficult than just stringing oneself along, but it is much less difficult. Cigarette smoking may be successfully discontinued very fast if one is honest with oneself and committed to the task.

41. If you're having trouble quitting smoking, go to a hypnotist for help. If you decide to try hypnosis, schedule an appointment with a licenced hypnotist. The hypnotist will put you into a deep trance and then repeat positive affirmations over and again in your head until they become permanent in your subconscious. It is likely that your subconscious will retain

these affirmations, which will aid you in your attempts to quit smoking.

42. Before you begin, you must be able to maintain your commitment to quitting smoking for life. When faced with major problems, far too many people try to leave on the spur of the moment and fail. Maintaining a high level of commitment is possible if you keep in mind the reasons why you want to give up. Modify behaviours that were previously linked with smoking in order to decrease smoking cravings.
43. Check with your supervisor to see if you can arrange your breaks at a different time to make it more difficult to give in to your cravings. Similar to this, if you've been smoking with your coffee all of your life, consider switching to a different caffeinated beverage like tea.
44. It is possible to assist your loved ones as well as yourself by quitting smoking. A number of malignancies, as well as a range of other health issues, are caused by secondhand smoking, which is very dangerous. In the event that you stop smoking, your family members will be exposed to less secondhand smoke, which will reduce their risk of health problems. Making the decision to quit will improve the health of you and your family. Steam should be released to prevent smoke being produced. When it comes to battling nicotine cravings, exercising is one of the most efficient ways. Another

advantage is that if you combine quitting smoking with an increased intensity physical activity programmer, you will see the benefits of your better health sooner rather than later.

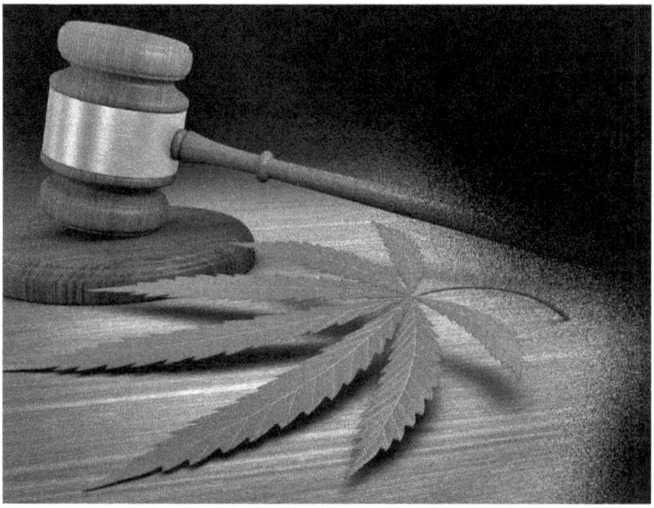

45. To successfully quit smoking, you must first develop alternate coping skills for dealing with the stress that you were previously able to manage by smoking, and you must avoid as many stressful situations as possible during the first few weeks of your effort. It is possible to deal with stress by listening to relaxing music, doing yoga, or receiving massage.
46. When trying to quit smoking, it is common for other behaviours that trigger the need for a puff to be modified as well. A glass of juice or water may be substituted for a cup of coffee or alcoholic beverage. After finishing a meal, many people find themselves craving a cigarette once more. After supper, take a walk. The fact that you are not smoking will not only

distract you from the need to smoke, but it will also help you maintain the weight loss that is often associated with quitting smoking.

47. It is essential that you put in place an appropriate incentive structure for such a difficult task.
48. It is essential that you put in place an appropriate incentive structure for such a difficult task. Treating yourself for at least the first three days and the first two weeks after quitting is recommended. Following that, you should commemorate monthly achievements until you reach the annual milestone. Furthermore, based on the length of time that has passed, you may choose your reward, making victory much more delicious.
49. Steer away from situations where you may be tempted to smoke, especially if alcohol is being served. If you find yourself in a party, bar, or other similar situation, it may be tough to keep your commitment not to smoke. If you drink alcohol, which lowers inhibitions, the task will be much more difficult.
50. Remind yourself that cravings generally subside in 10 minutes or less, so do everything you can to distract your focus away from the desire. Walk to the water cooler, have a healthy food, meditate, or talk to a supportive friend if you need to divert yourself from your need. This time will fly quickly, and your delaying

tactics may save you from succumbing to the temptations that await you.

51. If you can, try to view the benefits of quitting from a positive standpoint, as it may be very helpful to your overall well being. Taking this approach to decision-making will make it much easier to generate positive results in the long run. In order to stay motivated, keep in mind how important your job is and that the benefits of quitting outweigh the drawbacks. Keep yourself on track by acting as though leaving is an important matter.
52. Trying to stop smoking at a tough time in your life can improve your chances of succeeding. Attempting to quit at this point can only result in failure since your nicotine addiction is at its strongest. To leave, wait until you have gained confidence from previous successes, no matter how large or little, and then utilise that confidence to propel yourself out of your rut and into the world of work.
53. find out if there are any local smoking cessation support groups available by contacting your local health agency, clinics, or doctor's office. Interacting with other individuals who are trying to stop may provide helpful coping mechanisms as well as support and encouragement. If your friends and family members are not supportive of your desire to quit smoking, this may be especially helpful to you.

Epilogue

Marie struggled with controlling her urge and everything she did seemed not to be working at First. The motivation was there but she found herself slacking. She had the greatest support system anyone could ask for and they gave her their best. Her friendship with Charles was one of the mysteries she couldn't wrap her head around in, he was not embarrassed about her predicament and was not also ashamed of showing her off.

It was in one of their outings he introduced her to someone who finally became her partner in helping her achieving all her set goals.

After being sober for two years, Marie had decided to help other women going through the same challenge by establishing several AA meetings across the globe. She even organizes an online meeting and with the advent of technology, she sponsored many mobile applications geared towards helping alcoholic women. Charles was her strong ally and her partner in seeing this come to fruition.

Changing habits such as smoking, overeating, or drinking too much can take a lot of effort, and you may not make so much progress on the first trial. Setbacks and roadblocks are likely to arise, but with each experience and lesson learnt you get stronger. Each attempt will bring you closer to your set goals.

Whatever course you choose, give it a fair trial. If one approach doesn't work, do not give up, try something else. You will certainly stumble on one that works. If a setback happens, get back on feet as quickly as possible. In the long run, your chances for success are good.

Research shows that most people who drink heavily, even those with alcohol use disorder, either cut back significantly or quit. This is good news because there is hope.

CPSIA information can be obtained
at www.ICGtesting.com
Printed in the USA
LVHW020152020322
712401LV00007B/224

9 781915 322326